Man, Mind & Medicine

THE DOCTOR'S EDUCATION

A CHAIRMAN'S VIEW OF THE SWAMPSCOTT
STUDY ON BEHAVIORAL SCIENCE IN MEDICINE
23 OCTOBER—4 NOVEMBER 1966

Man, Mind & Medicine
THE DOCTOR'S EDUCATION

OLIVER COPE, MD

MASSACHUSETTS GENERAL HOSPITAL

With a Foreword by

ALAN PIFER

CARNEGIE CORPORATION OF NEW YORK

J. B. LIPPINCOTT COMPANY

Philadelphia & Toronto

THE SWAMPSCOTT STUDY on Behavioral Science in Medicine was supported financially by grants from The Carnegie Corporation of New York and the Commonwealth Fund. The opinions expressed are those of the author.

Distributed in Great Britain by
Pitman Medical Publishing Company, Limited, London

Library of Congress Catalog Card No. 67-30954
PRINTED IN THE UNITED STATES OF AMERICA
SP-B

Foreword

OCCASIONALLY CONFERENCES are held on subjects so intrinsically difficult, with such a high general level of discussion and at times such passion of debate, that production of the standard sort of report proves to be impossible. Such was the Swampscott Study of Behavioral Science in Medicine.

The following short book is, therefore, not a report but one man's view of the Study, that of Dr. Oliver Cope, its chief architect. And because Dr. Cope is himself a man deeply committed to the reform of medical education, a spirited advocate of an honored place for the behavioral sciences in medicine and, withal, a skillful writer, he has produced a document that, in my opinion, is of greater liveliness and value than any usual type of conference report could have been. It is of particular interest that a book on this topic should come from the pen of one of the country's most distinguished surgeons, a man who is on the staff of the Massachusetts General Hospital, and a professor at the Harvard Medical School. This book would not have been possible, of course, without the essential contribution made by the Study participants themselves. Their willingness to devote two weeks of their busy lives to this topic and the earnest attention they brought to bear on it deserve the highest praise.

Dr. Cope has addressed his book to the medical student because, in his felicitous phrase, the student is the "cambium layer of the academic tree." It is worthy of his attention, both for the immediate reasons given above and for the longer-range consideration that the enormous task of bringing the behavioral sciences into their proper place in medical education and the practice of medicine will fall on the next generation of teachers and practitioners as heavily as it does on the present generation. The Swampscott meeting was, indeed, only a beginning. As this book says, "The main work still lies ahead, in maturing

5

the ideas, reaching a consensus and formulating a workable program."

The task will be long and arduous. It involves not only a search for relevance in a world transformed by rapid social change, the same search which every form of professional education must make today. It also involves a basic reappraisal of the almost sanctified status of the hard sciences in medicine. In the more than half-century since Flexner, these disciplines have steadily been raised to the pinnacle of both professional and popular esteem, and deservedly so. But important as they are to medical education, they are not enough, and good as the practice of medicine is, it is not nearly as good as it could be. Its most serious inadequacy lies in its understanding of the social and psychological causes of disease and its general incapacity to take these areas sufficiently into account in diagnosis and treatment. The remedy is enhanced recognition of the behavioral sciences, and much greater attention to them, in medical education. There must be room for them too at the summit of esteem.

It is important for the reader to understand at the outset that the term "behavioral science," as it was considered at Swampscott, was by no means limited to psychiatry and psychoanalysis, or even to these two applied fields and their basic discipline, psychology. The term is, of course, and should be, much more extensive. For an adequately broad definition, I suggest an early look at the one given in Appendix B, the report of Dr. Beck's committee. Otherwise, the degree to which psychiatry quickly became the focal point of debate at Swampscott, which is reflected somewhat in Dr. Cope's account, may be misleading.

The study was jointly financed by two foundations, the Commonwealth Fund and Carnegie Corporation of New York. It comes as one important piece in a long-overdue reconsideration of medical education, which Dr. Cope and others associated with him are now, fortunately, stimulating.

ALAN PIFER
President
Carnegie Corporation of New York

October 1967

Contents

7

Prologue

REPORT OF A PATIENT

THE PATIENT, a woman, was 36 when she first consulted me in 1938. Born, bred and living in New York, she came to Boston to ask whether she really needed to have the hysterectomy and pelvic repair advised by her gynecologist. She had just been to him for her annual checkup. She felt well. Her catamenial cycle was regular, and she was not convinced by his arguments that she needed an operation. He had found her uterus a little enlarged and thought that she was probably building a fibroid. She also bore the scars of having had two children, a relaxed opening of the vagina, and an old tear on one side of the uterine cervix. The relaxed opening had given no symptoms, and he assured her that the old tear was well healed and without signs of incipient cancer. The gynecologist—a nationally prominent figure, Clinical Professor of Gynecology at one of the best-known medical schools—referred to the need for repairing the vaginal opening and removing the torn cervix as "tidying up," and she was shocked. Did these procedures really need to be done, she wanted to know?

Although this was the first time she had consulted me as a patient, I had met her once before. She was the sister of one of my college friends, and I had stopped at her parents' home in New York several times on my way to and from college. I remember seeing her when her first child was a baby and she was but 19. She had become engaged at 17 and married at 18, much against the advice of her mother. I had not seen her in the intervening 17 years, but I had heard of her periodically from her brother. He and I entered medicine together, and I had kept in close touch with him. I had formed the impression that she might have been a headstrong girl.

9

I had learned from her brother that after bearing two children—a girl and a boy—she had been through a harrowing divorce in 1931, while the children were still small. He related that she had been sharply critical of her husband, and that both she and her husband had been advised to seek psychiatric advice. This they did but the advice did not alter the course of events and they split apart.

Now seven years later, she told me that though the marriage had been tough the divorce had been a great mistake, and she longed for a second and successful marriage. The suggestion of a hysterectomy and the "tidying up" seemed to wrench away this dream and make a second marriage impossible.

On examination, she showed the signs of having borne children. The old tear of the cervix was well healed and there was no irritation. The uterus was a bit enlarged; presumably a fibroid had started. I told her that I could see no cause for alarm, indeed, no need to do anything at the moment. Fibroids are common enough and, for the most part, totally innocent; they are the bystanders and almost never the cause of trouble. I advised her, however, that since the issues had been raised, they could be solved by examining her periodically and waiting to see if anything untoward developed. She reported to me at intervals over the next three years. There was slight growth of the fibroid, no more than might be expected with the increasing years. Then came World War II; she changed her job and moved to another city.

One morning in 1944, she asked me on the telephone to see her right away. I saw her the next day. She was greatly perturbed. She had missed three periods and feared she might be pregnant. An obstetrician had found a much enlarged uterus, but thought it might be the old fibroid, not a pregnancy, and suggested that since I had seen her before I should know which it might be.

Her uterus was certainly enlarged, much larger than I had observed it previously, and easily the size of a midterm pregnant uterus. It also felt spongy and vascular. She did not show any of the other signs of pregnancy. I tried to reassure her about the pregnancy, saying I thought her fibroid uterus had suddenly become much enlarged and engorged. I then sat down and listened to her story. She had become intimate with a man much younger than herself, an old beau of her daughter. She found herself in love with him and he with her. She realized that the age difference was quite inappropriate and would prove embarrassing, but she hoped that they would be married. They had been having intercourse for some months, and although she had been taking precautions, she feared that they might not have been adequate. The consequences of a pregnancy would have been very distressing, and these had been on her mind for several months.

I suggested that her fear might well be a factor in missing her periods, and that we should do what we could to restore confidence. Fortunately, the pregnancy tests proved negative. As I learned more of her longings and of her realization of the inappropriateness of this love affair, I urged her to obtain better insight—in others words, to seek psychiatric help once again. This advice she steadfastly refused, although I thought I offered her substantial reasons each time I saw her over the next four years.

In the early months of those four years, her ovarian cycle returned to a normal rhythm. The boggy enlarged fibroid uterus shrank down to a half of the maximal size, and there it stayed until her menopause, which came in 1948 at the age of 46. Since then her fibroid uterus has peacefully shriveled to a slightly larger than normal postmenopausal uterus. No operation has proved necessary.

Another hurry call came seven years later. She had noticed that morning, before the mirror, that her thyroid was enlarged, and wanted to see me immediately. When she came to my office, she told me that six months earlier she had first noticed an irritation of both her eyes, a tearing and itching, a conjunctivitis unexplained by either her physician or ophthalmologist. The ophthalmologist had suspected incipient Graves' disease but her thyroid had been repeatedly examined and found normal. No enlargement was noted until that morning.

On examination, the thyroid was indeed enlarged and diffusely so, both lobes and the isthmus being involved. A bruit could be heard. Her eyes showed the changes characteristic of Graves' disease. They were more protuberant, and the palpebral fissures were wider than I recalled them. There was a lid lag and a diffuse conjunctivitis with tearing. The eyelids were a little puffy. In calm moments of our discussion, her pulse rate was normal.

The radioactive iodine uptake started that day was 77% at 24 hours. The BMR the next morning was plus or minus zero; previously BMR's had been in the low-normal range of minus 10.

She was obviously developing Graves' disease. The eye signs had appeared earlier, and now the thyroid enlargement had come on acutely and she would soon be in full-blown hyper-metabolism. How should she be treated?

The first thing to do was to determine, if possible, how this had come about. What were the etiologic factors? Could there be any explanation of why the eye signs had started first and then after so long a delay the goiter had appeared?

Again I sat and listened to find out what had happened. She had continued her relationship with the much younger man, and this despite no plans for marriage. She saw him only periodically now, because his business took him frequently to South America. She had, however, gone to spend a few holidays with him, and these had been most pleasurable and exciting.

Six months ago, he had invited her to go south to spend three months with him, but her mother, now well in her 80's, was ill, and she was torn. She had the premonition that this would be her mother's last illness. If she left on this pleasure venture to South America, her mother might well die while she was away. It was at this juncture that she first noticed her eyes. She went.

Her mother did die while she was gone, and she returned home to realize that she had never really made peace with her mother, and now it was too late.

All that her mother meant to her—her failure ever to have said this to her mother and her absence in the last days of illness when she should have been with her mother—had been brought home to her forcefully during the past several days, when she and her brother had come together in New York to close her mother's house and divide up the furniture and belongings. It was at the end of this emotionally searing task that she noticed her enlarged thyroid.

From the practical point of view of therapy, it seemed reasonable to assume that the emotional turmoil of the past six months had been the precipitating cause of the Graves' disease. The battle between pleasure and duty to her mother had presumably initiated the eye phase. The guilt over her mother's death while she was away on her pleasure venture, and finally the realization of what her mother really meant to her, were cause enough to have precipitated the second phase, that of the goiter. I already knew that her bodily organization was susceptible to disruption by emotional tension. These steps in the development of Graves' disease would be similar to the interruption of the normal ovarian cycle 11 years earlier from the fear of an unwanted pregnancy. But now her ovaries had gone to rest and that mechanism was no longer susceptible of being interfered with. The eye and thyroid mechanisms were perhaps next in line. At any rate, I took the chance and decided to treat her on the basis of the emotional tension, for this should reach both the eye signs and the thyroid enlargement. To treat the thyroid enlargement by one of the conventional methods would treat only that organ and leave the eyes unattended to.

I had of course another reason for selecting the emotional tension as the objective of definitive therapy. Forlorn and feeling miserable about her mother, she needed help. Childish ideas about herself still stood in her way. She felt lonely and was having difficulty making friends, indeed making any sort of intimate relation with people.

So I was firm, almost hard-boiled with her. I told her this was the time she must listen to me and must go to a psychiatrist, a psychoanalyst. She chose a well-known analyst and started on therapy immediately.

I did one other thing—and I don't know whether this had any effect, whether it should be given a share of credit for the subsequent course of events. Because her metabolic rate had not risen above an acceptable normal level, I started her forthwith on 180 mg of desiccated thyroid daily.

I saw her three weeks after the start of psychotherapy and thyroid medication. She was calmer and, curiously, her thyroid was less vascular and smaller. The thyroid medication was reduced to 120 mg daily. By six weeks, the goiter had miraculously disappeared. The thyroid gland was back to a normal size. The thyroid medication was reduced further, but because the exophthalmos had not changed, she was continued on 60 mg daily for the next three months, and then it was omitted.

The course of psychotherapy was by no means smooth. A year later, her analyst called me on the telephone to warn me about the severe depression she was in. The analyst feared possible suicide and, because the patient was going to be in New England for her summer holiday, sought my help to arrange some sort of guidance or supervision. Fortunately, the patient was successfully helped past this phase of depression.

I have seen her in late 1966. She is older; she now accepts her age, and doesn't attempt to appear 20 or 30 years younger than she is. She says that she is more contented and that she has built more of a life for herself. She certainly takes greater pleasure in her growing family. She has not remarried. At her last visit to me she said, "Look at me, would you ever know that I had those eyes and that goiter trouble?" I can still see a residual of the exophthalmos, but those who did not know her previously might not pick it up. Her thyroid has remained normal.

CHAPTER 1

Conduct of the Study

A PRESSING NEED OF MEDICINE is a better understanding of the role of behavioral science and of how to teach it. The role of the exact sciences in medicine is well established; research is flourishing and the teaching effective. Behavioral science, in contrast, has but limited acceptance; research is difficult and the teaching is less well organized. The study of the problems of behavioral science in medicine described in this monograph was carried out by a varied group of participants from college and medical school faculties and professional people outside of universities.

The reasons for the Study were many and various. Each participant had his own hopes for what it would accomplish, but the extraordinary acceptance of such busy people to devote two full weeks indicated how important they thought the subject to be.

All of the participants agreed that the behavioral sciences are important to medicine and constitute a major problem of the physician's education. There were differences of opinion, however, regarding what disciplines may properly be included among the behavioral sciences and which are important to medicine. Dr. Hamburg, Professor of Psychiatry, said:

> One aspect that seems reasonably clear to me is that there has been some confusion growing out of the fact that the conference was called "Behavioral Science in Medicine." I think it was no accident that the label was attached to the Conference. We are emerging into a period in which the study of behavior is clearly something broader than that which was associated traditionally with psychiatry. . . . It seems to me, and I say so with no shame at all, that this is one of the great frontiers in science even though it is exceedingly young and shaky. . . .
> I think we would all agree that the issues dealt with from the

15

medical and the social points of view are so important, the need for scientific understanding of these problems is so great, that behavioral science has to be pursued even if all of us in one way or another have misgivings about the adequacies of efforts to date.

Most of us would make the assumption—I certainly would—that in the long run, the more adequate the scientific basis of the underlying principles the greater the potency of the clinical judgment; but given the early stages of development of the behavioral sciences, I think that most principles best be viewed as highly provisional suggestions—which we utilize as effectively as we can at the present time, but which in a sense we can't take seriously, don't take as eternal verities.*

I agree with Dr. Hamburg's broad point of view regarding the behavioral sciences important to medicine. Two generations ago, psychiatry was the sole field of behavior taught as a part of medicine. As understanding has grown, it has become evident that psychology in all its ramifications is as essential to the understanding of psychiatry as physiology is to the understanding of pathology, the science of disease. Sociology and more recently anthropology have also joined the group of disciplines relating to human behavior and, along with psychology and psychiatry, are to be considered parts of behavioral science important for the doctor to comprehend. Disease, however, is what the doctor deals with, both in treatment and prevention, and when he cares for patients or looks at the mental health of the community he inevitably sees the problems from the point of view of the psychiatrist. This focus on disease can be narrowing; the doctor needs to keep in mind the breadth of the normal, the everyday, social and psychological forces impinging upon people, his patients.

Throughout the discussions came the question, how can this be taught? Is there a body of knowledge that can be taught?

The patient described in the Prologue presents a problem commonly met by the physician, a problem of bodily disease related in part to emotional imbalance. Such patients were in all our minds as we struggled with the questions of the Conference. Physicians differ as to how such a patient should be

---

* This statement by Dr. Hamburg is the first of many quotations from our discussions. The statements are taken directly from the recordings and in some cases have been edited by the speaker for clarity without altering the intent.

treated. The biochemical sciences have told us much about the physical nature of the patient's trouble, the psychiatrist something of the emotional disturbance. Physicians find it hard to correlate the behavioral aspect with the physical. Understanding of the total patient, mind and body, is fraught with uncertainties and is, therefore, an uneasy path for the doctor to take. He tends to follow the more certain path of the chemical sciences to the neglect of the patient's emotional problem.

No matter what the relationship is between the emotional and the physical, both have to be considered if the patient is to be helped. Few doctors have this capacity and few the feeling of responsibility for the family and the community. Present medical education too often fails to give doctors the insight and confidence that they need to handle both aspects.

Medical education is at fault. It is outmoded and needs an overhauling. An effort was made to start the overhauling two years ago at the Endicott House Summer Study.[1] In July of 1965, a group of professors, 34 in all, met at MIT's Endicott House to try to fathom what was lacking in medicine in the United States. They met with a sense of urgency, for much must be wrong. The country is short of doctors, and will be getting shorter. The character of medical care is rarely as good as it could be, and too many people receive none at all.

Professor Jerrold Zacharias, MIT Professor of Physics and member of the President's Science Advisory Committee, guided the Endicott House Study, fashioned on the pattern of his Educational Summer Studies. For eleven days, the participants hammered away at the problems, agreeing on a number of points. There was no doubt that the country was short of doctors, and it was agreed that new medical schools were urgently needed. Almost all recognized that medical education badly needed revision and that the new schools should accent experimentation in education. The new programs in schools and colleges provide more advanced students for the medical schools, and if the medical faculties were a bit adventurous, they could bring these students through the professional medical curriculum in three years rather than the present four, without loss of quality. The present medical curriculum is so crowded and so repetitive that one could only improve it by eliminating and shortening. More imaginative methods should substitute for the old lecture and laboratory system.

It was also thought that the graduate phase of professional education could be shortened—particularly if the young doctor started his practice as a member of a group, where he could continue to receive advice and supervision. It was recommended, therefore, that university teaching programs should experiment with types of group practice; that the universities should assume more direct responsibility for this graduate phase and for the new forms of practice.

The Endicott House Study did not have time to tackle the colossal problem of the behavioral aspects of medicine. Thus came about the Study known as Swampscott I, held at the New Ocean House in Swampscott, Massachusetts, from 23 October to 4 November, 1966. Knowing that there was no unanimity of opinion about the problems of behavioral science in medicine, the Steering Committee invited people of widely different backgrounds and points of view. It seemed important for representatives of anthropology, sociology, psychology and the arts and sciences faculties to bring their knowledge to bear on this problem. People were chosen because of interest and experience that would make them the foremost advocates of their points of view.

Jerrold Zacharias and his physics colleagues have sat down to their problems in an informal manner with free discussion and criticism. They have found that a prepared agenda tends to orient their thinking, and that it is better to allow the thoughts to come up spontaneously in informal discussions. With such a range of backgrounds, who could tell where the discussion might lead?

Following these lines of thought, the Study opened without an agenda. The first two to three days were presumably to be spent in working out the agenda, determining what was important, and then seeing how to go about it. The mornings and afternoons were taken up with much open discussion. Each evening there was a prepared program.

The participants formed a multidisciplinary, variegated group. First of all, there were four professors of medicine; as one might expect, they were well informed about behavioral science and the psychiatrist's role in medicine. They were Doctors Beck, Bondy, Leaf and Weisberger.

The pediatricians were Drs. Provence and Wedgwood. Dr. Provence, trained in psychoanalysis, was our expert in child development. Dr. Wedgwood pressed constantly for wider university involvement in the teaching of behavioral science and medicine in general.

The three surgeons, Drs. Child, Chase and myself were agreed that behavioral science is important in medicine. We differed, however, regarding the role of psychiatry—particularly the psychoanalyst—in day-to-day medical care.

Among the behavioral scientists, we had a remarkably rich and diverse group of representatives. Drs. DeVore of Harvard and Wallace of the University of Pennsylvania were the anthropologists. The psychologists were Drs. Hunt of Columbia and Shakow of the NIMH; Dr. Straus of the University of Kentucky was the sociologist. Dr. Kety from the NIMH represented the psychobiologists. Those forming the group of psychiatrists represented a wide range of points of view: Drs. Bibring, Coles, Quarton, and Stone, of Harvard; Bond, Lenkoski, and Rowland, of Western Reserve; Hamburg, of Stanford; Redlich and Solnit, of Yale; Snyder, of MIT; Tarjan, of UCLA; Eisenberg, of Johns Hopkins; Freedman, of Chicago; Barchilon, of Colorado, and Barondes, of Albert Einstein. Eisenberg of Hopkins was the most critical of the analysts' point of view—Barchilon and Bibring, the staunchest defenders.

Again and again, the participants looked to Charles Aring for a balanced point of view. He was our one Professor of Neurology; the psychoanalysis that he underwent as part of his original training in neurology perhaps accounted in part for his wit and balance.

Professor Zacharias had the vision to see that sooner or later we doctors must face up to the issues of behavioral science. He proved to be our gadfly. Hoping that we would be able to organize our thinking more to the point, more critically, he repeatedly tried to help us to focus on specific issues that we might be able to handle, and to avoid meaningless generalities.

We were not without support from the law and the humanities. Judge Bazelon, of the United States Circuit Court of Appeals, listened intently, sought help from the psychiatrists, and by striking comparisons with the law helped clear our vision. In like manner, we were assisted by James Dixon, physician turned college president, and by Reed Whittemore, who drew his examples from the teaching of English, and Roger Katan, who used his experience with programs of urban development. Several times Professor Langer, historian of Harvard University, pointed out to us how we were off the rails in our historical conclusions.

Between periods of discussion came presentations by several visitors, and motion pictures made by biologists and anthropologists. Professor Hans-Lukas Teuber, of MIT, described his observations in neuropathology. Dr. Count Gibson told of his experiences with the medically deprived poor, of Columbia Point in Boston and the Delta in Mississippi. Dr. Robert Coles brought three bright Harvard students of the third year class— men who had been involved in the insurrection the year before during the course of microbiology, when 25 students asked to run their own course, rebelling against the crowding and repetition in the medical curriculum. These students described to us also the coldness of the courses and a lack of contact with patients and thoughts about human behavior.

From the very beginning, the meeting was never at a loss for someone who was willing or eager to present his views. Almost immediately the chairman started the practice of writing on the blackboard the names of those who wished to speak. To give you an idea of the vividness and intensity of the discussion, when the more debatable points were under discussion rarely less than seven people waited their turn to comment. Occasionally the discussion was heated.

By the end of the fifth day, we were bogged down on two or three questions, and it seemed wise at this point to break up into smaller groups to see whether we could make better progress. Accordingly, we divided into groups, each chaired by a professor of medicine. Insofar as possible, participants representing special points of view were divided among the committees. Periodically, the committee of the whole met to hear the progress of the separate committees or groups. There was no set program for any group. Here again, each group was urged to follow its own interests and thoughts, and, as one would expect, the written comments from each group differed considerably in what they thought was important and how the situation was to be met. The discussions of the committees were not recorded, but a written report from each group is in the Appendices.

The atmosphere engendered by the Zacharias approach is far different from that of the customary medical conferences; they usually have a prepared agenda. Many, and sometimes all of the participants, have been assigned a subject to present. Having been given this responsibility, they rarely assume a comparable responsibility toward any of the other subjects. They have an obligation to rebut or answer any comment made about their own subject, but they may assume none for commenting on the others. Indeed, more often than not the program is so full that there is little or no space for commenting, and what few comments are made have often been assigned beforehand. The conference is completed in double-quick time, in, say, two or three days. The prepared speeches are pulled together in some kind of publication, the whole is published, and that's it.

What is needed, of course, is to have the participants so involved that they cannot escape, so interested that they insist on expressing their point of view, and will consider, perforce, the views of others. Thus in the end they will be ready to take action.

With this thought of eventual action, the Steering Committee left the meetings unstructured. No arbitrary limit was placed by the chairman as to the angle from which the idea was to be viewed or the degree of criticism and discussion to which it was to be subjected. With issues as important as those we faced— involving the human being, his thinking, his emotional balance, his actions—no limit could be placed on debate. Two weeks seems like a long period, but it was considered almost certainly too short by Jerrold Zacharias. The diversity of opinion made this abundantly clear. The two weeks were but a beginning; the main work still lies ahead, in maturing the ideas, reaching a consensus, and formulating a workable program.

Because behavioral science is an area essential to the advance of medicine, and because only a few teachers have found thus far a way to teach it well, the Steering Committee decided to address this monograph to the student—for many reasons.

In the first place, there is evidence that many students undergo an undesirable change in their point of view toward medicine and, in particular, toward behavioral science. Most students come to the medical school open-minded and free to consider all aspects of behavior and science important to medicine. Something happens during their four years. The educational mold distorts their vision in such a way that they become increasingly centered on the exact sciences to the detriment of their interest in the behavioral and emotional aspects of the patient. The participants at the Conference felt that this must be brought to the student's attention, so that he will be on his guard.

It is essential for him to see, then, something of the significance of behavioral science before he becomes overwhelmed by all that he has to learn. The requirements for entry to medical school are long in the exact sciences, and his educational experience in college, therefore, tends to have been long in the hard or exact sciences. There is no objection to this, provided he doesn't think that it is the only aspect of medicine that is important. The college experience, however, tends to make it easier for him to follow the chemical aspect than to delve into matters foreign to his earlier education. It is important for him to know that he must honor equally the exact sciences and the behavioral sciences. It is also something for the faculty to pay attention to, for it is difficult for them to see. Faculties are highly specialized; the chemists, the anatomists, and the pathologists are busy with their daily tasks and their researches. Their minds are on their own disciplines, and it is natural that faculties should be slow in becoming aware of areas outside their own field.

The material of the Study has been divided clearly. The second and third chapters describe the problems encountered in patients, how the doctor sees them and how he handles them; the second includes the everyday behavioral problems, the kind all doctors should recognize, and the third psychosomatic medicine, an area requiring the special knowledge of the psychiatrist.

Though the physician can learn to deal with patients suffering from psychosomatic disorders, he needs special training.

The psychiatrist is the subject of the fourth chapter. The participants disagreed as to what kind of person he is or should be. The fifth chapter addresses the student himself, and considers the special things that he needs to pay attention to. It is based on the assumption that he is mature and prepared to assume responsibility for his own education. The sixth and final chapter concerns the obligation of the faculty to the same problems.

Behavioral science was not the sole area left without adequate consideration at the Endicott House Summer Study. Closely allied to behavioral science is the problem of women in medicine, and this has two aspects: numbers of physicians, and the character of medicine. Some think of encouraging women in medicine to supplement the number of doctors and in this manner to help relieve the shortage of physicians. The second and more important reason for the admission of more women to medical schools, however, is to encourage women to have more of a voice in the character of medical practice. American medicine is still a man's world. Medical students, men and women, are pressed through the same rigid educational mold. The women graduates compete in a man's market for internships and residencies. Women are discounted for surgical residencies because it is feared that physically they may not be able to maintain the pace set by the men. No thought is given to what a woman's special insight and intellect might mean in the care of the patient with uterine bleeding or a lump in the breast. The male is impressed by the ease of removing the uterus or the breast. Would a woman surgeon, encouraged to independent thought, advise otherwise? Were she to write a text on the diseases of women, would it be the same as those now available, all of them by men? There are also reasons beyond the diseases of women suggesting the need for more women in medicine; these include the upbringing of children and the social aspects of medicine generally. Women in medicine, therefore, will be the subject of a subsequent study.

A third study, the second sequel to the Endicott House Study, was held at Swampscott, April 23 to 30, 1967, and has dealt with the graduate phase of medical education. The graduate phase, the internship and residency, is perhaps the most important and at the same time the most knotty. It is important because the graduate program sets the precept for the undergraduate; the resident sets the image for the student. It is knotty because somehow the practical aspects of caring for patients have to be learned and tested. The phase is, therefore, intertwined with and dependent on patient service. Not only new thinking, but some experimentation is needed. The universities must assume responsibility. The Swampscott Study is but a start. The idea that the graduate phase of medical education needs attention is also not new. The Coggeshall Report of April, 1965, and the Fort Lauderdale Meeting of February, 1966, dealt with it, and most recently the Millis Commission of September, 1966, urges reconsideration and experimentation.[2, 3, 4]

The Steering Committee and the author in particular wish to acknowledge the support of each of the participants. They at one time or another contributed all of the thoughts described in this monograph. We also thank Dr. Stone and Dr. Barondes for their special part in keeping track of the deliberations.

The Committee would also like to acknowledge the enlightened support given by the Carnegie Corporation of New York and the Commonwealth Fund in the organization and conduct of this study.

The author was enormously helped in the sorting out of the ideas of the Study, and in the arrangement of the monograph, by Mrs. Ruth Hapgood of the Houghton Mifflin Company, and is grateful to Miss Rose Setterberg and the other secretaries for their conscientious care of the details of the Study and the final preparation of the manuscript. To Mr. Kevin Smith and others of the staff of the Education Development Center, we also extend our many thanks for showing us their superior motion pictures and for their recording of the Study.

CHAPTER 2

Medicine's Need for Behavioral Science

GENERAL PATIENT CARE

THE PROBLEMS OF BEHAVIORAL SCIENCE may be divided, like all Gaul, into three parts: first, those common problems of patients, the concomitants of their physical troubles, which all physicians encounter and handle of necessity; second, those problems of patients needing the special knowledge of the psychiatrist; and third, the problems of community mental health. Mental health is an issue little appreciated and still scarcely touched on in present-day medical education. Although mental health and the social implications of mental health to the community were many times referred to during the Study, time did not permit their full consideration. An essential part of preventive medicine and all-important as it is, mental health will not be mentioned further in this monograph.

The patients whose problems stem wholly or in part from emotional and psychological difficulties need, in general, more expert management than that of the general physician, unless he has had special education and experience. This is the realm in which the psychiatrist is needed, and it is considered in Chapter 3.

The present chapter deals with the problems of the first category—the emotional and behavioral troubles frequently encountered. They range from worry over enforced idleness to the realities of dying. All doctors encounter them, ophthalmologists, urologists, internists, and all the others. For the most part, they have not been an etiologic factor in the disease which the patient suffers.

Everybody, well or sick, has an emotional side, both conscious and unconscious. Like an automatic pilot or governor, it guides a person through his life. In the sick, this guide may be well-balanced, helping the patient through his illness, or it may be far off balance, a hindrance to his progress. It is the business of the physician to seek out this balance in every patient and to know which way it is acting. Some good physicians do this in-tuitively; many others of us have to learn how. But it can be learned.

I am not talking about politeness; I have nothing against it. And I do not mean warmth or a slushy sentimentality. I am talking about the practical gains in patient care which stem directly from the physician's awareness of the emotional side. Sick, worried people are highly sensitive to a doctor's interest in them. When they sense that the doctor is not interested in them as persons but only in the so-called scientific aspect of their trou-ble, they become reticent, freeze up, and do not divulge mate-rial which may be important in reaching a proper diagnosis and directing effective care.

The gynecologist who recommended the hysterectomy and "tidying up" to the patient of the Prologue lost her confidence by his failure to realize what a hysterectomy would have meant to her desire to get married. Had he listened and tried to put himself in her shoes, he would have been less likely to advise what subsequently proved to be an unnecessary operation. Had she known no other doctor to turn to, or had she had something more serious, such as an incipient cancer, her loss of confidence in him might have had an altogether different consequence.

What are some of these common problems? Eventually all people die, and one of the commonest problems facing physi-cians is, therefore, death. At the present, no accepted way exists to handle this age-old problem; it is treated on a hit or miss basis.

The subject of death was introduced by Dr. Wedgwood. Sev-eral hours were spent in discussing the fear of dying, the special problems faced by the patient in a terminal illness, and the ways in which the physician may help the family and friends of the dying. The discussion was presided over with restraint and wisdom by Dr. Aring, who has long given special thought to these problems.* Many of the participants contributed. Below I quote two telling examples, verbatim, as Dr. Solnit recounted them. A third example is one of my own, showing a pitfall into which I fell through ignorance and unawareness. A fourth and fifth are cited by Dr. Bond. Several of the participants joined in the discussion.

Dr. Solnit: We have been much concerned with teaching students and house officers in pediatrics about the dying child and trying to learn something about this ourselves. One of our earliest experiences indicated to me that the intensive study of the individual, comparing the individual to himself at different times and in different situations, provides a scientific method for such clinical studies.

One experience involved a 45-year-old man, who had a very early adenocarcinoma of the kidney removed successfully, it was thought. But a year and a half later, he was referred for codeine and morphine addiction to the psychiatric clinic. I thought he looked very sick physically. We had another film, which had not been thought necessary, and we saw that a snow storm of metastases had broken loose. The urologist, at that point, felt that his ward was unable to cope with this dying patient, so we took him on as a patient at the Yale Psychiatric Institute, to be cared for by the doctors, nurses and social workers in the Psychiatric Hospital. He died in the Yale Psychiatric Institute. Initially, there was a lot of raising of eyebrows; why was a patient who had such a malignancy dying in a psychiatric ward? This man was followed very carefully and taught a number of us many things. For example, he kept telling us, in many many ways, Don't tell me I am dying. He kept saying, Don't keep me away from my family, so his family was in a great deal; and he also said, Don't keep me away from my medicine. Incidentally, he was not addicted to morphine. He was addicted, if you want to use that term in the figurative sense, to the fear that no one would pay attention to him. He was afraid that no one would pay attention to him if he didn't have pain. He was terribly lonely. He was frantically afraid of being alone.

In working with children, one of my most vivid experiences involved a little girl, who asked me, "Could you tell me what this leukemia is?" I asked her why she wanted to know. She said, "I know I have it, but everyone around tells me I am not supposed to

* Dr. Aring's remarkable insight into death and care of the dying is given in his "Intimations of Mortality: An Appreciation of Death and Dying," a lecture given at Western Reserve in September, 1966.[5]

know about it." She was 11 years old and she read, watched TV, and listened to her doctors and parents. It isn't only the denial on the part of the patient that one must assess but our own need to deny both health and illness, the need of parents to deny, the need of nurses to deny. Some denial is very helpful because, as Ernest Kris once said, if something is intolerable and insufferable, the best thing you can do is to deny it. Then there is the amount of denial with which this little girl was being confronted, and she was saying, "I know I have got leukemia; I don't want to know all about it, but I would just like to know a little something about it."

For the sake of visual representation, I would suggest a triangle on the blackboard. You would have the patient; you would have the doctor and the helping people, teachers or whoever they might be, and the family, friends and community. They are involved in a complex situation, the center of which is the patient, who is dying, who is trying to cope with this as another one of the problems of the end of life, which is my way of saying what Dr. Aring said so well. Our aim is to help the patient, family, and medical team to master or cope with the dying process, and not to be overwhelmed by dying or death.

For children, three fears are involved: the fear of somatic pain; the fear of helplessness, not knowing what you are doing and what will happen next; and finally, what I would call the fear of loneliness, of being alone. These are the critical reactions that are universal for the dying child. If there is one common motivation for people being in medicine or in the healing arts, it has to do with the interest in warding off the destructive forces accompanying death.

Dr. Cope: When I was a fourth-year student, William Sidney Thayer—the great professor of medicine at Hopkins, that wonderful understanding warm human being—came to Harvard and gave a *Care of the Patient* lecture. He described malignant disease and told how you handled it and how you always had to tell the patient the truth. This was a vivid experience for me. He described a patient who had come to him in Baltimore because he had been put off by physicians elsewhere. He knew he wasn't getting the answer, and so it was easy, I suppose, for Dr. Thayer to know that the thing to do was to tell him. The patient wanted it; that was why he came to Baltimore. So he told him. The fellow, of course, was upset; and his wife was angry with Dr. Thayer. He said she berated him: "What right did you have to tell him?" Then, two hours later, he got a telephone call. They had gone back to their hotel, and called Dr. Thayer to thank him for having told, because for the first time in several months, the two of them could sit down and talk.

That was a vivid model, and now I think of my mistakes. A woman had obvious cancer of the thyroid, and knew it. She knew it because of the way her physicians dodged telling her; everybody was alarmed. Any fool could see that her doctors were alarmed; so she made me promise the night before the operation, religiously promise, that I would tell her the truth. She suspected the truth; she outlined to me the number of reasons she needed to know. She was a widow; her children were not quite launched and so on; and I had to tell her for very practical reasons. So it was. It was a rapidly growing, undifferentiated carcinoma, the type with a wretched prognosis, perhaps nine months or a year, and it would have to be treated by radiation.

So I waited until she was over the anesthetic, and the next morning I came in, pulled up a chair next to her, sat down by her bedside, and said: "I will now do what you asked me to do. You have a serious condition: we are going to give you x-ray treatment. There is no doubt that these treatments will help you. It is possible we will manage to eliminate the trouble completely, but just the same you had better do what you said about rearranging your estate and taking care of your children and so on." She thanked me very much, and I went out with great relief, thinking that I had carried it off. In the next two or three days, I was congratulating myself because she had taken it so well; I must have done a good job. On the fourth postoperative day, the nurse stopped me before I entered the room. "You know, Mrs. B is waiting. She wants to know when you are going to fulfill your promise and tell her what you found." I was younger then than I am now; I failed to take advantage of the broad hint offered me by the patient, namely, that she had shut out the bad news. So I went in and I said, "I hear from your nurse that I haven't told you. Don't you recall that the very day after operation I told you?" "Told me what?" So I went over it again. She, of course, went into a serious depression; and it was terrible. It ruined her life and, what is more, mistakes seem to be contagious. To make a long story short, the pathologist and I thought this was an undifferentiated carcinoma. It wasn't: it was one of those very peculiar tumors. The same type of tumor was found in the wall of her stomach four years later. She lived for 12 years after that to die of a coronary.

Most of us doctors don't have the understanding to manage these situations and we badly need to learn how.

Dr. Zacharias: Can you conceive of any kind of formal education that would have helped you with that?

Dr. Cope: Yes, something, but certainly not what I had had. I acted on the single model given me, persuasively, by Dr. William Sidney Thayer.

Dr. Eisenberg: Did you ever watch him do it instead of being told by him how to do it?

Dr. Cope: No.

Dr. Weisberger: You don't really teach a doctor to do this; the patient will do it if you let the patient tell you. Cope's patient tried to do it by saying "You didn't tell me." It is just like showing the laws of a pendulum.

Dr. Bond: I don't know that it is formal education, but I think it enormously helpful if somebody who has had some clinical experience in this area says to the student, "Now listen to this talk and let me show you." The patient has all the things that make it easy to show this kind of denial. If you say to the student this is the proper thing to observe, usually it is such a loaded and such a surprising observation to a young student that he can't forget it. For instance, I was up on a medical floor one day when a young colleague of Dr. Weisberger received a hurry call about a patient on the floor. The colleague was very upset because it was a woman medical student who had lupus. The technician said, "I went in there to do something and the medical student patient said, 'What are you doing?' " She said, "I am doing an LE prep; gosh, why did I say that? I have told." The 'phone rang and the nurse said, "Your medical student patient wants to see you right away." I told the physician, "Don't worry, I will give you $5 if she mentions anything about the lupus. She is going to tell you that the window was open, the food was lousy or that the nurses hated her." So he went down there, the food was lousy, and that was it. She never made the slightest mention of the lupus. He remembers it because he paid me $5 for it. The point is that the patient chooses. She denied to herself that she had the lupus.

A man wrote *I Have Cancer*. It was picked up by the *Reader's Digest*. He got 400,000 letters from people from all over the world saying it is marvelous to tell us the truth. By this time, he had lost 150 pounds, was being transfused every other day; and as his physician was leaving, he said, "Doc, what are my chances?" The doctor, taken very much aback, said, "Only a miracle can save you." He went into an hysterical reaction. Some other people got into it and they asked him to be a scout for the rest of us because he was going to the land beyond. His friends and wife also became hysterical and got the bright idea that cancer was psychosomatic and that a psychiatrist should treat him. I got the wife aside and said, "Look, this man is almost dead; will you let him die like a man. Please keep your neighbors out and you remain calm. Let the man who lived like a man die like a man." I would go up and see him, and he would tell me what happened to him when he was four. I would say, "That was marvelous, I will see you Wednesday night." Wednesday night, he would tell me what happened when he was five. "Fine, I will see you Friday night." Finally, he died quietly. But it is simply amazing that a man like this who had lost 150 pounds and been transfused countless times turns to you every other day and says to you, "What are my chances?" The power of denial is very strong indeed.

Question: What should the doctor have said to him?

Dr. Bond: I think the doctor did as well as he could.

Question: The doctor said only a miracle could save him?

Dr. Zacharias: I don't blame the doctor at all for that.

Dr. Solnit: It is an impossible question. You can't answer the question that way, what is the *right* answer? You have to say what the answer is that a particular doctor would give a particular patient.

Dr. Redlich: On what is his information based? What does it go back to? What has he learned that he could do? Is it something that he just knows because he is a very broad man? That is what interests me.

Dr. Zacharias: I don't see how you get any grip on any of this.

Dr. Leaf: It seems to me if we are going to be talking education, then the question when we deal with this particular problem is, Is there a body of knowledge available to be transmitted to students, or is there not? If there is not, can we sensibly set up studies that will give us some information?

Dr. Eisenberg: The point of this story, it seems to me, is being missed. In a word, it is that the physician cannot make the correct decision for a particular patient by using himself as the touchstone; that is, judging how the patient is feeling by how he would feel if he were in the same situation. What the physician must keep in mind is the range of human behavior and that a question or a complaint is likely to mean more than it says. It is useful to lecture to or discuss with students human reactions to death, and to give them some vicarious experience by citing illustrative examples. This will, to some extent, prepare them for what they may see when they confront the first dying patient, and help to protect them against being overwhelmed by the experience. Discussion with others and gradually accumulating experience of their own will enhance the student's skills and effectiveness in comforting patients. Dr. Weisberger has acquired a background of experience and personal sensitivity. A good internist with these attributes can offer the student a great deal of help. I would emphasize that this is empirical help and does not require that we have a comprehensive theory about reactions to death. I am not decrying theory, but I am pointing out that the sensitive physician can help the patient and can teach the student to help the patient even when his knowledge is incomplete.

Dr. Bibring: I would like to answer Dr. Zacharias and Dr. Leaf somewhat differently. There is a body of knowledge available to be transmitted to students. It is not only the work of intuition, but the result of systematic studies of personality types and the kind of defenses patients apply against trauma and anxiety. This can be taught and learned.

No routine solution is satisfactory. There is no overall rule that will be of help to every patient alike. Under the trying condition of terminal illness, it seems of special importance to know more about the patient, to differentiate between personality types, and to adjust communication and medical management to the different personality diagnoses. There will always be patients who feel safest and best taken care of if they can leave the knowledge of their condition in the hands of their doctors, without having to face the truth fully by themselves, and there will always be patients who will have to know whatever there is to be known about their illness. Otherwise patients in this latter group, once they suspect a serious diagnosis, do not feel safe with their doctor any longer and do not feel they can trust him fully. Between these two types, there is a variety of others, each of which deserves our full attention in order to achieve the best possible result.

Mutilation, particularly that involving sexual function, is another common problem encountered by physicians. Yet it has been considered almost not at all by those surgeons forced to practice it. Psychiatrists and an occasional physician are well aware of the emotional turmoil that many patients are thrown into by such mutilations as hysterectomy, mastectomy, orchidectomy, and radical prostatectomy. They understand something of the part the surgeon's personality may play in leading the patient to accept and subsequently manage the deficit, but rarely does the surgeon himself understand, and in his literature little of authoritative nature has been written.

The following account was written by a patient with cancer of the breast. This cancer is the commonest cancer afflicting women and the second commonest cancer known in the total population. Radical mastectomy has been the traditional approach to the management of this cancer for more than 50 years, yet I know of no article in the literature—by surgeon, physician or psychiatrist—dealing with the emotional consequences of the threat of losing the breast.

My surgeon has asked me to write as directly as possible what I experienced when a lump was found in my right breast some months ago. I, like most other women, had been instructed to examine my breasts regularly to prevent just this emergency. This I had done from time to time, imagining that I did it regularly, so that when during a routine physical examination my medical doctor found a lump in my right breast, my reaction was one of disbelief rather than dismay. It could not be serious. It must just have started. Nothing to worry about, but what a nuisance.

My doctor's suggestion that I should see a gynecologist did not increase my anxiety. His manner reassured me; he didn't seem worried. The gynecologist examined me carefully and he too identified the lump in my breast. His expression sobered. I should have a biopsy he said; the tumor was probably not malignant but should be checked immediately. This I knew was reasonable. I would have, I imagined, no more than the bother of a minor incision, a few days rest, and the incident would be behind me. He suggested that I see a younger man who, he said, did this operation, which he himself no longer performed.

The younger doctor went over my breasts, my neck, my armpits. Then he stepped back. Yes, there was a lump there and I should have a biopsy to determine what it was. Probably it would be benign, but one could take no chances. And I should have it done as soon as possible.

Well, there it was. I had better find out what was entailed. My husband and I were to leave in four days. How long would the biopsy take? If it were positive, how long would I be laid up? Would he please tell me exactly what to plan for?

Underneath the straightforwardness of my questions I was experiencing a mounting concern. Would it be cancer? Would I lose my breast? Inconceivable. But, then, the first operation, a biopsy, would be a minor one and should there be a malignancy, I would have time to prepare myself for the more serious operation and its consequences.

A biopsy? Well, this was done while the patient was under the anesthetic. A frozen section was made, and if this should show any malignancy he would proceed to remove the breast at once. Remove my breast, he said. I would go to sleep not knowing and wake up ineradicably altered. Forever. I pressed on, frightened now and angry, determined to know the worst at once in order to deal with it.

"You never do a biopsy first and then an operation?" No, they did not. "Why not?" Well, it was unnecessary to go under the anesthetic twice; easier to do it all at the same time. "Will you take more than the breast?" Well, sometimes, he explained standing there in front of me, it was necessary to remove the glands under the arm, and sometimes even the muscle underneath the arm. And then there would be radiation therapy afterwards to insure that there would be no spreading of the malignancy. "But my arm! It's my right arm! How much will I be able to use it afterwards?" He hesitated. Well, there would be almost normal use, he said, but perhaps the up and down forward movement would be slightly impaired. It would be almost normal.

Almost normal! What was he talking about? Take off your breast, cut out your muscles, and then assure you that you would be almost normal. I was furious. I looked at his young, calm face, and I thought You don't know, What conception have you of what this means? It's just the way it is always done. The way it has been done for years and years. Surgeons always want to tidy things up, anyway. I knew I was not being reasonable, that cancer was a fearsome disease, but at this moment of anguish the cool objectivity of his attitude struck me as being less than humane.

The next few days are a blank. When I told my husband, I made as light of the whole matter as I could; it would be only a minor operation and surely the tumor would be benign. Whether or not he believed me, he helped me by pretending that he did.

But my anxiety overwhelmed me. In the night, I awoke shaking. I would go back to my doctor and tell him that this was impossible, that there must be some other way. It was indecent to be caught like this with no alternatives. It was inhuman. I must be able to act in my own behalf, and make a reasonable choice. I understood now why women, when they found a lump in their breasts, refused to go to a doctor, refused to save their own lives. Rather dead than maimed. (It was never as conscious a choice as this, I suspected, but these were the roots of the delay.) Foolish, short-sighted, ignorant, perhaps, but deep down the intense desire to preserve one's own identity in physical form, to keep one's own life.

It still seemed incredible to me that there should be only one solution, with research going on all the time, impossible that the answer should still be no different from what it had been for fifty or more years. I would go to my doctor and see if he would help me.

Busy as he was, he showed me into his office and listened to my story blurted out rather incoherently. I was on the verge of tears. "If it could be more gradual," I told him, "first a biopsy and then the larger operation if it were necessary. That is how one does with plants. One acclimatizes them to changes in temperature and situation so that they will not die. Can't people be treated as sensitively? Or are there too many of us? Can't human beings be treated as other than bodies?" He looked at me sympathetically from where he sat on the other side of his desk. "Now, don't feel bad, dear. It will be all right." And that was it.

To add to my worry, I found out that my gynecologist did operate on patients with breast tumors but perhaps not on friends. I am his friend and neighbor. Is he avoiding me because my tumor is serious?

The following day the papers, which I was to fill out, came from the hospital. A night's sleep and resolve guided my hand on the page. My name, my address, my Blue Cross number. Did I want a television in the room? Slowly I filled in all the blanks. Plenty of women had this operation and survived very well. If they minded the loss of their breast or their arm muscles, they didn't say so. They stepped along as proudly as ever. Why was I making all this fuss? So what did it matter if you had only one breast? Probably your husband would not mind. Probably. Probably you would get used to it, even to the look of the scar. The scar, what did it look like? No, you would never get used to it. Never. You would just endure it. What lousy luck. I signed the paper.

That night, tossing in the darkness, an alternative came to me. I had a surgeon, a friend who had concern for me as a person. He had operated on my thyroid years ago, and when I had been threatened with a hysterectomy had given me good counsel and helped me to avoid it. He would perhaps help me this time.

My husband went with me to his office high in the new hospital building. Warmly he greeted us. My dossier lay on his desk. "Sit down," he said, "and tell me how you have been since you were last here." He listened quietly to what I had to say. "Suppose we see what is there," he said, "I should be very glad to take care of you."

Again the examining room, but what a difference. Already my confidence was rising, quite irrationally. With deft and skillful fingers he examined my breast. "Yes, you do have lumps, not one but several," and he showed me small, very small points under the surface of my breast. "How could I not have noticed?" I wondered.

When I had dressed, I went again into his office. He sat at his desk, hands folded. "Let me tell you what I do," he said. "I first operate, remove the tumor and do a frozen section. But I do nothing more surgically. I do not remove your breast. What I do is to treat the cancer with radiation therapy, first under your arm and the entire breast and then on the other side of the breast on the front of your chest. This prevents the spread of cancer without surgery. You will not have changed at all physically. You will be the same as ever. The radiation therapy will take about six weeks. You will have to be careful of being in the sun for some time afterwards, but that will be all. This, I believe, is just as effective a way of dealing with such a condition."

Later, I was to understand all the whys and wherefores, when he explained to me in detail the sound reasons why he found that this method of treatment was preferable to the other, and why ten years ago he had adopted it, and how statistically the results were the same, perhaps even a little better than when radical surgery was used. But at the moment, all I could feel was the intense flood of relief and gratitude that surged inside of me. I would not lose my breast. I would not be disfigured. I would have full use of my arm. I need not undergo a prolonged recovery, and never, never need face myself in the mirror with the right breast cut off. I was rescued.

The study made no attempt to discuss in a comprehensive way the numerous other emotional situations that the physician encounters day after day. For example, neither hysterectomy nor breast feeding was discussed. Doctor Redlich described the undesirable consequences that may result when a patient asks a physician who is a close member of the family to assume responsibility. Several other models of behavioral problems in this area were offered, but death occasioned by all odds the most intense attention. No one was able to provide the formula for the care of the dying. It was left in the realm of intuition, a subject each student should become aware of, and one certainly in need of study. Dr. Aring felt that all students should at some point be involved in the care of a dying patient, that this is at present the best way to alert him and help him teach himself.

Doctor Weisberger reminded us repeatedly that all physicians must learn to deal with these common problems. There never will be enough psychiatrists to go around to care for the patients with such problems. Besides, many of the situations have to be met immediately and the psychiatrist would be arriving too late too often. These problems of behavior constitute, therefore, a major issue of medical education.

CHAPTER 3

Psychosomatic Disease: Need for the Expert

THE PATIENT OF THE PROLOGUE suffered two bodily diseases, irregular uterine bleeding and exophthalmic goiter. Some physicians consider both conditions to be generated at least in part by psychological turmoil. Psychosomatic disease is the term now generally accepted to mean this special causative relation of disturbed mind to physical disorder. Although all physicians may agree with the definition of psychosomatic disease, many hesitate to acknowledge its existence in recognizable clinical entities. Few agree to the list of diseases to be included in the category, and still fewer are prepared to use the concept in the treatment of the patient. Such lack of agreement existed among the participants of the Study.

Agreement regarding the etiology of the psychoses and severe neuroses is also lacking. Some favor genetic and biochemical origins; others see emotional influences or factors of environmental origin. Although these diseases fall within the orbit of behavioral science in medicine, a stage beyond psychosomatic disease, they will not be considered in detail. They will be referred to in the next chapter about psychiatry.

On the afternoon of the fifth day of the Study, a discussion of psychosomatic medicine evolved out of the following interchange between a participant and Judge Bazelon:

Participant: In medicine, you have to include all the enterprises we are talking about. This is the view that society now takes of it, and I don't mean the Gross book[6] on how awful doctors are. I mean the television Dr. Kildare attitude that we can do everything and, as the Judge said a little while ago, if we keep at it, we are going to be running society.

I have changed my mind about a number of things in the last few days. We are going to get so overextended we may lose our capacity to educate people. Society thinks that our job is to make everybody happy who isn't happy, and this has been alluded to. You people [psychiatrists] have been quite candid and said you don't know how to do this either. The people out there think this is what we in medicine do, that we make unhappy people happy.

Now in medicine, and I think this applies also to the surgeons, our primary job is to keep people from dying earlier than they ought to die, and to keep them from having painful and incapacitating disease. If we learn how to do that, that is a very demanding, exacting thing. I tend to downgrade what we have accomplished in the last 20 years. But, I predict that in a couple of decades, most of the major problems are going to come under some kind of control. This is big important work, and we ought to keep at it.

If it is possible to train people to cope with unhappy people, whether they are mentally ill or just unhappy, outside a medical school, we better get to work and learn how to do it real fast. We are not going to train enough psychiatrists from the medical schools to staff these mental health clinics unless we use only the psychiatrists who have had mental breakdowns; and medical schools aren't going to make it any other way. You can't staff those things with the products of the American medical school now or ever; and someone else is going to have to enter the field. I am not sure I am all for lay analysts, but I am all for lay people who are wise, educated and understand something about behavioral science and know how to listen to people and give them some guidance in their lives. I don't think medicine can carry this job.

Judge Bazelon: Then I have one question. I speak from an abundance of ignorance when I ask: Aren't there many diseases, heart disease and other things you are talking about, that do have some psychological basis or overlay?

Participant: That's been overstated; I don't really believe it much.

Judge Bazelon: If you don't believe it, you should have said so at the onset of this meeting.

Participant: It's been exaggerated a great deal.

Judge Bazelon: Then you should have said we don't need the psychiatrist.

Participant: We don't need a psychoanalyst to tell us how to cope with the psychological problems of a fellow with a coronary thrombosis. You just need to know how to treat patients with that disease.

Judge Bazelon: There are some people here who feel that there may well be a psychological genesis, at least in part, which you can't ignore.

Participant: It isn't the cause of cancer; it isn't the cause of heart disease, and it isn't the cause, I don't think, of strokes.

Judge Bazelon: Not strokes?

Participant: No.

Judge Bazelon: I don't know on my own, but there is disagreement. What if they convinced you otherwise?

Dr. Bond: I think you would have a hell of a time convincing him otherwise.

Participant: I think that psychosomatic things became very fashionable a decade and a half ago, but now it's all immunology and I don't know what it will be next.

Dr. Bond: For instance, I think any one of us would say that there are certain concomitants of emotions that are physiological and that these can have at certain times rather remarkable effects on various parts of the body given other circumstances—something like that. I suspect everybody would agree to that at least. How you go about it and how you view it may vary a little bit, but in general, psychosomatic medicine is not as fashionable now as it used to be.

Dr. Quarton: It would be unfair to put it just in terms of fashionable, though. The psychosomatic model has broken down partly because it is based on a naive notion of cause and effect. If you think in medicine there is one cause and one disease, that is silly. It is a little bit like dealing with the host factors in bacterial disease. If you are really interested in psychosomatic disease, then you have to understand the way in which environmental factors acting through the brain and through cephalic processes alter the physiological function of the body, and how that interacts with other causes of disease. That's a perfectly relevant field of research. It happens to be very difficult, so that some of the people who are interested in a little harder science have slowly been leaving this field because they want simpler and more manageable problems; but as a medical phenomenon where you need methods of care, this is still a perfectly relevant field.

Dr. Bond: Dr. Cope, we gave you a rather backward introduction to psychosomatic medicine. Do you want to comment?

Dr. Cope: I welcome the opportunity.

Dr. Quarton is right in objecting to the use of the word fashionable. Diseases are not fashionable, but treatments may be. There is no evidence that psychosomatic diseases are less common than they were a decade and a half ago. They may be less publicized, and physicians may be less aware of their existence because the treatment has not been as simple and effective as was hoped 30, 20, and even 10 years ago. Dr. Quarton has suggested some of the reasons. The original thoughts and conjectures about psychosomatic disease were overly simplified. In recent years our understanding has expanded rapidly. Precision has begun to emerge. The original concept or conjecture of an emotional factor in psychosomatic disease is amply sustained.

Psychosomatic diseases abound. They are to be found in relation to almost every organ of the body, and if migraine headaches can be called a disease, then the brain itself is to be included among the organs.

Judge Bazelon was correct in sensing that several of the participants knew that many conditions had a psychologic genesis, at least in part, and that these conditions cannot be ignored. Perhaps it is right to exclude cancer as a disease in which there is a psychologic component. To my knowledge, none has thus far been identified, and from the life histories of the cancers we know well this doesn't seem to be a likely place to go looking. It is wrong, however, when it comes to heart diseases and strokes. Laymen know better than this. There is more than one form and one cause of heart disease, but the lay know that losing your temper or worrying excessively with loss of sleep are just the conditions to bring on an attack of paroxysmal tachycardia, a myocardial infarction, or a stroke. We don't need a physician to tell us this.

Dr. Quarton's statement is important because it points out that there are multiple factors—the psychological or emotional only one of them. Because all of the factors are by no means understood, Dr. Zacharias has suggested that we use the term "contingency" rather than factor. I like his amendment.

The brain manages all bodily functions. It runs the cardiovascular and pulmonary systems. The heart and the lungs have no brain of their own to tell them what to do. The function of these two organs is enormously complicated. For example, messages from the periphery, from the limbs or the intestines, pass to the brain telling of a need for blood. In response to these requests a host of adjustments need to be made about cardiac output, cardiac rate, blood pressure, and blood distribution. The flow of blood has to be coordinated with the respiratory system, and that in itself is no mean trick. Only the brain could do as well as this.

The same sort of thinking holds for digestion. True, a built-in minor endocrine system helps digestion, but this endocrine system is supportive, not primary. The primary control of digestion is seated in the brain. That is why the operation of vagotomy has some use in treatment. The vagus nerve does not start an inch or two above the diaphragm, where it is handy to the surgeon, but stems from the medulla oblongata, and that in turn is controlled by centers higher in the brain stem. This simple anatomy is the reason, I suspect, why the Russians have once again been emphasizing the work of Pavlov.

The brain also controls the major endocrine gland system. In Cushing's time, we were taught to think of the anterior pituitary as the bandmaster calling the tune, balancing its function off against the gonads, adrenal cortex, and thyroid. Now we know that the anterior pituitary is at most the concertmaster or only one of the first fiddles. The pituitary is subservient to the brain and not infrequently is by-passed in the system.

This recent knowledge regarding the brain's control of endocrine function at first sight is surprising, but the basic mechanism has been known for a long time in regard to the secretion and release of the oxytocic and antidiuretic hormones.[7,8] These two are secreted in the supraoptic nuclei of the hypothalamus and pass, in the neural pituitary stalk, into the neural hypophysis, where they are stored but not secreted. They are released by a nervous stimulus.

As long ago as 1932, A.S. Parkes showed that ovulation in the ferret was controlled by the hypothalamus.[9] Since then, in every mammal in which it has been investigated, ovulation has been ticked off finally by the brain. In most, the final stimulus comes from coitus, and the effect of the brain can be prevented by dividing the pituitary stalk. Although it is not proved in the human being in the same way as in other mammals, there is reason to suppose that the same conditions exist in woman.[10] Nothing so important to the survival of the species as ovulation could be left to two spineless glands—the anterior pituitary and the ovary—to lob it back and forth across a net.

The anterior pituitary is still viewed as an intermediary in the control of several of the glands—namely, the thyroid, the adrenal cortex, the islet tissues of the pancreas, the gonads, and perhaps the thymus. The mechanism of control in these systems is now believed to be as follows.

For each glandular system, there is at least one control center in the brain, probably in the hypothalamus; additional centers may be elsewhere in the brain. These centers are comparable to the supraoptic nuclei secreting the posterior pituitary secretions. The centers have been identified for some of the systems in a number of animals, but they are poorly understood still in the human being.

The hypothalamic centers are believed to secrete what are now called Releasing Factors.[11, 12, 13, 29] These factors have been named the Thyrotropin Releasing Factor, the Corticotropic Releasing Factor, et cetera. The factors pass into the portal-hypophyseal circulation, a venous system that flows down the outside of the pituitary stalk and bathes the glandular cells of the anterior pituitary in a portal-like circulation.[14] The anterior pituitary cells respond by secreting into the general circulation the specific trophic factor—the Thyroid Stimulating Hormone (TSH) for the thyroid, ACTH for the adrenal, and the various gonadatropic factors for the gonads. The growth hormone also is believed to be secreted in response to a similar mechanism, though the center for the control of growth has not as yet been identified. Biochemists have identified a large number of these releasing factors.[12] They are polypeptides, chemically closely related but with highly specific actions.

Less well understood is the control of the hypothalamic centers. However, important experiments indicate control from elsewhere in the nervous system. Two surgeons, Hume and Egdahl, have demonstrated that the adrenal cortical hormone is released into the blood flowing from the adrenal cortex of a dog as soon as five minutes after the dog's hind leg is burned.[15] The effect of the burn can be cut off by transecting the spinal cord above the afferent nerves from the limb. If then in that animal the forelimb is burned, the adrenal cortical response is again observed. In an animal in which the cervical cord has been severed, there is no such response from a burn to the forelimb. In this type of preparation, Egdahl has obtained evidence that there is also a center for the release of the corticotropic factor in the brain well posterior to the hypothalamus.

Experimental neurologists have presented evidence showing that the limbic system contains centers inhibiting the hypothalamus.[16] If the influence of the limbic center is removed, the hypothalamic center acts at a much higher rate. Thus the limbic system might be compared to the thermostat regulating a house furnace. If the thermostat is cut out, the furnace goes on burning and the house is overheated. This is the state comparable to hyperthyroidism. The temperature-regulating mechanism of a mammal placed in a cold environment, say in a refrigerator, calls for an increased output of thyroid hormone. Placed in a warm environment, the output of thyroid hormone is reduced or shut off. There is evidence that the temperature-regulating mechanism of the human being exercises a comparable control of the thyroid output.

Because the brain runs pretty much everything, it would be amazing if the mind when disturbed did not result in bodily changes and bodily troubles. The evidence that psychological turmoil may be a factor in the eruption of physical disease rests largely on clinical observation. Evidence gained from experimental animals, though suggestive, is not too helpful. Laboratory animals are apparently difficult to upset, perhaps because they have so little mind. Gastric and duodenal ulcers as a sequel of stress in the executive monkey have been found in one strain and not in another.[17] Genetic susceptibility is therefore an additional factor. A rise in thyroid function has also been shown under the executive type of stress in another strain of monkeys.[18]

Farm animals abound in endocrine disturbances as the result of a kind of social stress. Egg production of the common domestic hens is lowered or temporarily stalled by moving the hens from one house to another. The milk production of cows, likewise, is reduced by moving them from one barn to another, or from one herd to another. A mare may be finicky, and the surroundings must be just right for her to ovulate and conceive. In contrast, the ovulation of the cow is rarely disturbed, so that impregnation is easily accomplished by bull or artificial insemination.

Now to the clinical evidence for psychosomatic disease. I have had more experience with Graves' disease than with any other. It was in 1943 that Dr. Stanley Cobb, our professor of neuropathology, pointed out to me that it was high time that we of the Thyroid Clinic began to look into the psychological aspect of Graves' disease. For some time I floundered around, not understanding what he meant and unable to come up with anything substantial or utilizable. Little by little, however, I have come to see many things.

First of all, the patient who develops Graves' disease was not an emotionally well-balanced person to begin with. This observation is obtained usually by history, but sometimes patients have been observed by an interested physician prior to the onset of the endocrine disorder. I have had this opportunity several times myself. Second, comes an added, acute distress. This ticks off the endocrine disorder.

Three things are important about the psychologic components, the supposed psychogenic factors of Graves' disease: first, the predictability of the presence of the components; second, the variable character of the components; and third, the need for expertness in their understanding and management. Regarding the first, the more skeptical participants asked repeatedly whether there is a predictability about a supposed situation like this. In my experience, there is.

Since I have learned the trick, when I see a patient with Graves' disease I just wait until the patient describes the precipitating situation. The patient is able to do this with predictable regularity. It is as Dr. Weisberger has said—just let the patient talk. The event or sequence of events is usually vivid and tormenting to the patient if the disease is of recent origin. More difficult for the patient to describe is the psychologic background that one might say had sensitized the patient. This aspect is usually buried and professional skill is needed to uncover it, more skill than I have for the most part.

From patient to patient, however, the psychological turmoil is by no means always the same. This is the second point. Both the factors in the background and the precipitating situation are variable. Lidz and Whitehorn, in describing the psychologic factors of Graves' disease in 1949, thought that they had found a quite comparable situation in the 16 patients they examined.[19] I am unable to agree.

I shan't take the time here to document the predictability or the variety of situations which may give rise to hyperthyroidism. Jerrold Zacharias has pointed out that perhaps the reason why psychosomatic medicine is not understood better by the medical profession is that we have failed to document the situations so that they are evident, learnable and convincing. Documentation is tedious, but I agree with Dr. Zacharias that it should be sharpened wherever possible. Accordingly, I am documenting elsewhere this statement regarding predictability.[20] An important aspect of this documentation will be the evidence for the other factors or contingencies, especially the endocrine and the seasonal.

The several doubters among the participants questioned the predictability of the cure of bodily ills by psychotherapy, and I have dwelt on Graves' disease because it is a condition for which relief by psychologic means is predictable. Psychotherapy is also more comprehensive and therefore better than the traditional treatments. Operation, RaI, and the antithyroid drugs attack only the thyroid gland, the end organ of the disease. They leave the emotional component unattended to, and this may go on to produce progressive exophthalmos or in later years some other bodily disturbance.

Two final points: the more promptly the patient is helped to see the psychological situation, the more prompt the relief; and second, not all patients are able to take advantage of psychotherapy. The very situation in which they are trapped prevents their seeing the need.

Cushing's disease seems to me to be so like Graves' disease in many of its aspects that I have little doubt that Cushing's disease, too, is a psychosomatic disorder. Comparable emotional backgrounds and trigger mechanisms have been found with such regularity that they are now predictable in patients with adrenal cortical hyperplasia. (This I shall also document in an article to follow this monograph.) Some cases of essential hypertension and duodenal and gastric ulcer appear to be psychosomatic and with predictable psychologic aspects. When I have taken the time with these patients, each time I have found a plausible situation. This is a sort of unsupported guess, a hunch.

Drs. Weisberger, Beck and Bondy did not share the reluctance of some participants to accept the evidence regarding psychosomatic disease. These three felt that I was making much ado about nothing in arguing. To this, I point out that I've seen in consultation patients with Graves' disease from many areas of this country, usually from university hospitals or university faculties. Many professors of medicine and surgery don't seem to understand psychosomatic disease, and if they think they do, they give it but lip service. As an example, a young doctor's wife with Graves' disease was referred by a professor of medicine at a medical school two thousand miles from Boston. She was anxious to avoid the operation that had been recommended. I told her perhaps it could be avoided if she could tell me how her disease had come about, and provided that she and I could reverse the situation. She was prepared for this statement because she had been reading everything she could lay her hands on, and had come across a chapter I had written on this subject. At her next visit, she confided to me the tough situation in which she was trapped. Tears flowed down her cheeks. She felt that this had much to do with why she was sick. I then asked, "Did you not tell Dr. So-and-So about this?" She answered, "When I first saw him, he asked me whether I had anything on my mind. I was not prepared for the question and before I could gather myself to respond he went on to the next question." This professor of medicine gave lip service to the emotional aspects of her troubles. He is a conscientious person, but obviously he does not understand. Dr. Weisberger should take him in hand.

The trend in practice today is to expect chemicals, the tranquilizers, to solve these problems and to feel that psychotherapy is not needed. For the patient whose situation precludes psychotherapy, tranquilizers obviously may be better than nothing, but for the patient who can be reached and within whose capacity it is to alter the irritating circumstances, tranquilizers are but a temporary shortcut. This too, I shall document.

A university colleague, a friend of many years, turns to me from time to time for medical advice. Six years ago he underwent a major orthopedic operation, and was helped through it by a distinguished cardiologist and an equally distinguished internist. Since then, he has been seen with some regularity by these two physicians. Recently he has noted a feeling of tightness starting at the back of his neck and spreading to the head.

It feels as if his blood pressure were rising. The tightness comes on when he is under particular stress. In addition to his university duties, he is an internationally known figure and bears a heavy responsibility as an adviser in international affairs. These bouts have come in recent months when he worries about his responsibility to the Vietnam War. The internist has prescribed tranquilizers. The reason my friend called me is that he finds the tranquilizers do no good and he senses that the problem is beyond the internist and the cardiologist. He says frankly that they don't understand. He is perceptive enough himself to realize the probable origin, namely, that he has taken on more than he is able to handle, the responsibility is too much, and there are acute phases in the pressure. He wants to know what I think he should do. He would like reassurance from his physicians that there is physically nothing wrong; he feels that this is all he can ask from them. If this is true, then he must try to handle his responsibilities himself, since neither of his doctors is wise enough to appreciate the problem.

As I view it, there should no longer be any argument about the existence of psychosomatic disease and the importance of dealing with the psychologic aspect. For the moment, the best the nonpsychiatrist clinician can do for a patient with these troubles is to determine if there is a psychological problem. This may take some doing and we may, therefore, need the psychiatrist to teach us how. As to treatment, successful lasting improvement has called for the expertness of the psychiatrist.

CHAPTER 4

Psychiatry and the Psychiatrist

THE POSITION OF PSYCHIATRY in behavioral science, medicine and medical education was argued over at length throughout the Study. In many parts of America, the psychiatrist is still not accepted with grace as a full partner in clinical medicine, least of all the Freudian analyst. Although the psychiatrist is turned to on every hand to care for patients, including members of doctors' families, progress in his acceptance by medicine is slow. Although there is improvement here and there, and many successful psychiatric units have been organized, opinion among physicians and among behavioral scientists ranges from strong support to severe condemnation.

By good fortune, the various points of view regarding psychiatry were represented among the participants of the Study. On almost all aspects, there was disagreement, divided, however, not according to disciplines. Among the clinicians, for example, internists disagreed with internists, surgeons with surgeons, even psychiatrists with psychiatrists. Among the nonclinical scientists, the anthropologists and psychologists, there was also no unanimity of view regarding the role of psychiatry in behavioral science.

All of these points of view have been recorded in the literature, and extensively. Why have they not been ironed out? Why has the psychiatrist not been accepted generally as a partner in research as well as in clinical care?

Six Issues

The issues raised are divided, for convenience, into five: psychiatry as a science, the effectiveness of therapy, the time required, fees, and the language used. The author has added a sixth, the criticism.

PSYCHIATRY AS A SCIENCE

The following is a forceful statement of some of the criticisms of the psychiatrist.

I think I would like to be quarrelsome. It may be useful to say some unpleasant things now rather than just sit around for ten days nodding at everyone else and having them nod back. We are a mixed bag of people in this room, we have very sharp differences of opinion here, and I think it useful to get them out into the open so that we understand how far apart we are from each other. I can speak freely about this because I don't think I am going to hurt anybody's feelings.

I hope we don't begin drawing diagrams, trying to do what you want, Zacharias, which is to get a case from which generalizations can be made. This is the trouble with psychiatry from the prejudiced point of view of people in internal medicine. I think this is what psychiatrists have been doing ever since Sigmund Freud. Their literature consists of paper after paper on a single case, with all of his dreams, from which immense theories are derived, and they do draw diagrams endlessly.

The question must be raised whether psychiatry is in any sense a behavioral science; and if it is a behavioral science, is it the science basic to the clinical problems our medical students see in the third and fourth years?

I think medical education lacks a behavioral science serving the needs of psychiatry in the sense that physiology and microbiology, to some extent, serve the need of medicine as a discipline. I don't think the "basic science" offered by the conventional Psychiatric Department, as it is taught in the first two years, has a lot of meaning and certainly doesn't have anything more than a religious content.

Now there are scientific things going on in the behavioral field that are extremely interesting, but they are going on in the universities, for the most part. People are working with animals on such things as autonomic conditioning of rats, or deprivation phenomena, or the influence of crowding, or the inheritance of instinctive, very complicated patterns of behavior. Medical students don't hear—at least at the schools that I have seen—enough about these matters at first hand. Behavioral science is a proper fundamental field for all of medicine, including psychiatry. But psychiatry itself can no longer pose as its own basic science.

I shall make one more, sort of irritating, point. At many of the medical schools in this country are what are called analytically oriented departments in psychiatry; and they turn out fellows—some of them even won't put white coats on their house staff for fear the fellow will look like a doctor—who spend the rest of their lives in a peculiar relationship to money, as if it were part of therapy. They even charge our medical students when they break down. No other person on the faculty or in medical practice would dream of charging a fee to a medical student, but psychiatrists, with great regularity, charge whatever it is, $25 a week, when an occasional student has felt such a need. Another unexplained attitude of some psychiatrists is that they have really left the field of medicine—and I am not sure that they ever belonged in it in the first place. For instance, I don't know what the difference between a lay analyst and a medically trained psychoanalyst is except that the medically trained psychoanalyst has had by and large an inadequate training in medicine. Most of them have one year of internship, usually a rotating internship. They are forbidden to take more than this one year, and you can't learn much medicine in this way. It seems a kind of a waste of everybody's time.

I don't really mean all these things, and I am not sick. I think they have to be said by somebody to get us underway.

Dr. Leaf conceived of the role of behavioral science as bringing humaneness into medicine.

Dr. Leaf: First of all, I think all of us would agree—maybe I better be careful about saying that here—many of us would agree that one of the attributes of a good physician is that a physician has to be a warm, concerned individual with empathy toward suffering people.

Dr. Leaf stressed, indeed, that social and behavioral sciences were important to medicine and that they should be included in the curriculum of the medical school, but he questioned whether analytic psychiatry should be included in these disciplines.

Dr. Leaf: I would think that if there are these areas where the social and behavioral sciences can help us do the job the community expects of us, then we may put down the disciplines that Dr. Wedgwood mentioned must be considered in our medical curricula. I think whether analytical psychiatry gets included among these disciplines is an open question, in my mind, but there is a lot here that can be discussed.

Dr. Leaf called attention to criticisms frequently leveled against psychiatry, namely, that psychiatrists depend too much upon the anecdotal approach and that in their research they do not use standards of control comparable to those of the scientific disciplines of medicine.

The position of analytic psychiatry in medicine and medical

education was most staunchly defended by Dr. Barchilon, who told us how reproducible and satisfactory the formulations of analytic theory are. Dr. Barchilon started his medical career as an experimental neurophysiologist with Walter B. Cannon. It was Dr. Cannon who suggested that he explore psychoanalysis. As a scientist, he was much impressed with the reproducibility of the formulations and theories. He illustrated his points with two brief case reports of the anecdotal type objected to by several of the participants.

Dr. Bibring, one of Freud's pupils, presented the case of a young hysteric to show how the analytic concepts may be used in teaching medical students how to examine the emotional aspects of a patient's illness. She emphasized in this case report the predictability of aspects of hysteria. From the analytic point of view, the hysteria was classic and Dr. Bibring's presentation historic.

Dr. Redlich took a more moderate position.

I don't think anyone can present a unitary theory of behavior. If you asked the people in this room to agree on a unitary theory, you would not get agreement. We have only segments of knowledge, which have to be fitted together. Is a unitary theory indispensable? Internal medicine doesn't have such a theory. They have bits here and there, and in this respect, psychiatry is not worse than internal medicine. It is, as a matter of fact, like internal medicine, not a science but an application of sciences. All of us probably believe that a certain scientific knowledge about behavior exists and is relevant for the practice of medicine. The question is what is this knowledge. It includes, in my opinion, bits of knowledge about development, learning, social systems, culture, communication, ethology, and most of all, unconscious motivation. No super theory is necessary: it doesn't exist anyhow. The next question is, How to teach this knowledge to medical students in an interesting and relevant way, and who should teach it?

A week later, he had the following to say:

I have little bits of feeling, and they are pretty much that we are back where we started. We make some progress and then like a cursed ship in the *Arabian Nights,* we must have sailed back again to the same point. We could talk about psychiatry, whether it is an advanced glorious field, whether it is a primitive field, whether it is—as Derek Denny Brown once said when I was on his service— 90% common sense and 10% Germanic nonsense, or whether it is a real field. I personally believe it is an emerging field; it has basic sciences.

Dr. Eisenberg was highly critical of the dogma of psychoanalysis, but he was exasperated with what he considered the unreasonable criticisms.

I find it quite unreasonable that several of the participants display intellectual arrogance toward work about which they know next to nothing, and I mean that literally. I would not try to pass myself off as an expert on renal or infectious disease, even if I had had a chance to read the literature. There is, even if you may not know it, a considerable body of factual data on mental illnesses. There are highly developed and very sophisticated methods and theories in behavioral science. The fact that there are many areas of ignorance in psychiatry (or that some psychiatrists are ignorant) does not mean that nothing is known.

Dr. Zacharias sought a way of bringing the points of view together.

I believe the people here are not communicating with each other. They are talking past each other; they are doubting each other. *Until they come to grips with* some facet, with some piece of psychiatry that can be looked at in every way, they are not going to communicate with each other. Second, I believe that what we have missed in every psychiatric presentation is a clear analysis, psychoanalysis, of what was in the psychiatrist's mind, all of the things he discarded, all of the things he went through very fast, or sometimes slowly, the alternatives and whatnot, so that you can see what kind of combination of experience and discipline the psychiatrist was trading on. I am sure the experienced psychiatrists in the room have been through this enough so that they know it; but for those people who have not done it in that way, and this includes some of the people who are physicians and not psychiatrists, and for those of us who have not done it in this particular way as a profession, there must be, I think, an exhibition of this.

On the following day, Dr. Zacharias had this to say:

There isn't any one of these things that has any sharp boundaries or edges. If you go trying to get people to agree on sharp boundaries and edges on something that is foggy, I think you are wasting time.

The historian comments.

Professor Langer: It seems to me what I hear people saying here is that the so-called hard-nosed medical scientists recognize that they need something more. Call it behavioral sciences in general, psychiatry in particular, and so forth; but they don't like the behavior of the scientists and psychiatrists whom they see around. They say that they are not doing hard-nosed research, that they are not analyzing things in the laboratory, and that this is not really science and we had better not get mixed up with it at all.

Judge Bazelon had still another point of view.

As you have been talking here this morning, I can't help thinking about what we call our common-law system. Some of you here, I am sure, must be familiar with it. The genius of the common-law system is that it requires constant reexamination. You have a case, say 50 years ago, on which the information and understanding of that day were applied in order to reach what men then thought a just solution. Now what happens is that someone seeks to apply that decision to a case 50 years later. But the controlling effect of the earlier case may be vitiated by new information and understanding —a different context, if you will. Now that is what we are supposed to do, and that is exactly what we fail to do too many times. We just take the principle of the earlier case—or precedent—and apply it without regard to the new context. You talked today about teaching the student. You seem to be searching for a principle that you won't have to reexamine—apparently because reexamination is too complicated, too difficult. You seem to be looking for a system that works without difficulty like an automatic machine operation—a system of self-executing principles, so you don't have to get involved with your own guts. Now we have this problem in law. Too many lawyers talk pridefully about the dynamic concept of the common-law system, but in practice they abandon the process of reexamination and adhere to a static concept with its illusion, or delusion, of certainty. I am suggesting that you may be looking for principles, to hand to the medical student, that will obviate the necessity for getting his guts involved in the decisional process. It seems to me that it is a futile search.

Dr. Shakow and Dr. Hunt were upset by the vehemence of the arguments among the clinicians regarding the disciplines of psychiatry and psychoanalysis. Dr. Shakow has recorded his thoughts in a separate report (see Appendix F). Dr. Hunt had this to say:

I don't think that most of you have any idea of the impact of our discussions here on someone who has been trained in psychology as a discipline and who doesn't want to be a junior doctor. A lot of things have been said that rock a person like Dave Shakow or me.

Psychiatry seems to have been taken as the basic behavioral science for medicine. Psychology, as such, has hardly been considered, even though it has content and flavor quite distinct from psychiatry and psychoanalysis. Somehow, sometime, what is *actually in* psychology should be looked at in these discussions of behavioral science in medicine. There is a whole series of amazing things that happen in psychology.

Dr. Hunt stressed that clinical psychology is a science to be pursued for its own sake. It is also useful to medicine because of the knowledge it has already amassed. He continued a few minutes later.

Dr. Hunt: The clinical psychologist, if he would retain his identity and stick to his lab, would have a great deal to offer because he gets the culmination of things that none of the others do. What happens is that he gets into the therapeutic situations and he finds he is doing therapy. I can, if I wanted to, lose my role; I could spend all my time applying what is known already to the problem of drug addicts and alcoholics; there is a big enough bag of tricks so that I could be busy the rest of my professional life—thoroughly distracted from the much more fundamental issue that psychotherapy and behavior change are not going to be produced by a series of animal training devices, which in effect will teach a patient to do something different—just as we teach a seal to play "God Bless America" on the horn.

The specialties in psychology that have trapped themselves in the medical model have become sterile intellectually, and exciting new developments in the science of behavior have had to arise in other quarters. Actually, close working relations between medicine and psychology could and should be fertile, and there should be interfaces with many medical specialties in addition to psychiatry.

The problems of human illness can stimulate basic investigations and challenge current knowledge. Similarly, the results of psychological experimentation so stimulated can enlighten medical practice and add to psychological theory. This will not happen, however, if psychologists in clinical settings yield to temptation and lose themselves in medical identifications.

A frequent criticism of psychiatry as a science is that although Freud was a great figure, nothing has happened since Freud, no important discoveries or advances have been made. As I view the history of psychiatry, there have been many advances in understanding. Painstaking intelligent researches are going on in many areas of psychiatry, from neurophysiological observations in brain localization to the interpretation of dreams. One might say equally that there has been no advance in bacteriology since Ehrlich. In 1910, when Ehrlich announced the discovery of salvarsan, he had formulated the theoretical basis for antibiotic chemotherapy. All the modern antibiotics are consistent with his original thesis. Do the modern antibiotics represent no advance? Eisenberg is right. Those who criticize the science of psychiatry have not taken the time to inform themselves properly.

EFFECTIVENESS OF THERAPY

The second criticism leveled against psychiatry is that its therapy is uncertain; and furthermore, that there are no reliable methods of appraising the results of treatment.

In examining the criticism that psychiatry does not seem to benefit the patient, one has to ask what kind of patient, what kind of mental disturbance. Psychiatry is limited in what it can do for schizophrenia and manic-depressive disease. These are the cancers of the mind, and it is surprising that psychotherapy ever achieves anything with this severe type of disorder. Yet, curiously enough, it sometimes is able to achieve relief, perhaps never cure, but certainly remarkable relief. The same internists and surgeons who level criticism against the psychiatrist don't do very much for their patients with comparably severe diseases. The physician who cares for the patient with nephritis may by intelligent management tide him over an acute phase, but is able to do little himself about the primary disturbance. Survival of the patient depends upon forces beyond the physician's control. The surgeon is almost without influence upon cancer of the stomach and is lucky if 25% of his patients with carcinoma of the breast survive the disease. The physician and surgeon who utter this criticism of the psychiatrist lack humility.

If the criticism is leveled against the psychiatrist's care of patients with anxiety and noncrippling emotional disorders, the type of disturbance leading to psychosomatic disease, then the criticism to some extent is reasonable, for certainly with some patients the result of psychotherapy is uncertain. The methods of appraisal, like the science itself, are not sufficiently developed to be certain. But to say that results are not proved because no valid methods of appraisal exist is to fly in the face of abundant experience. The good physician who has tried to help his patient by simple reassurance and, having failed, has turned to psychiatrists, has repeatedly learned what the psychiatrist's special knowledge can do for that patient. Certainly continuing research is needed in developing possible methods of appraisal, but as the science advances, these methods will become automatically available.

It is the patient himself who knows best whether he has been helped by psychotherapy. The critics of psychotherapy point out that the quack also helps patients. True. But there is a difference in character between the relief given by psychotherapy and that induced by the quack. The benefit induced by quackery rarely leads to sound physiologic reasoning by the patient, and the benefit is short-lived, as in all placebo treatment. The benefits from psychotherapy, on the other hand, are associated with an improvement in the understanding and reasoning of the patient, who is usually able to recount the evidence for his improvement in understandable psychological terms.

It is helpful to visualize whence much of this criticism of psychiatry comes; I have met this criticism from various types of physicians. It comes from certain professors of medicine and surgery who have had almost no contact with modern psychiatry. Some of those professors manage services in large general hospitals where no well-rounded psychiatric service is available to them for consultation. The only psychiatrists available are those caring for the patients with psychoses, overloaded with the patient burden of city and state hospitals. These professors in medicine and surgery have no working contact with psychiatrists skilled in recognizing and dealing with the subtleties of personality of everyday people.

Other medical professors who have had contact with sensitive, effective psychiatrists yet who continue to inveigh against the unscientific nature of psychiatry, have just not given sufficient thought to the nature of man's psychological processes, their subtleties and vagaries and the limitations these peculiarities impose on scientific study. Their evaluation involves judgment, and judgment is not measurable in the same finite terms possible in physics and chemistry.

Still other professors are obviously resistant to pyschiatry. It may be that they are made uneasy by examining emotional content of patients. Surely they are not lazy. They avoid psychiatry, or make light of it; some even ridicule it, a firm indication of their uneasiness. They don't ask for psychiatric consultations for patients on their wards or for their private patients; they have not visited the ambulatory psychiatric clinic of their own hospitals; often they don't know who cares for the patients in these psychiatric clinics. They are often people who "don't dream," in other words are unaware that they dream, and think of the psychiatrist's interpretation of dreams as a sort of Mephistophelean quackery. They have avoided examining the modern developments of psychiatry and count on chemical understanding of nerve function to yield all the answers.

In regard to dreams, they have been unwilling to see that the analysis of a dream can today be as important to a psychiatric evaluation of a person's problem as the examination of the urine is to the physician wondering about possible nephritis or diabetes mellitus.[21-25] Modern recordings of electroencephalograms and rapid eye movements during sleep, together with the description of dreams afforded by the patient when he is awakened, indicate beyond peradventure that people dream though they may not be aware of it. If the patient is coached to become aware and perseveres in remembering his dreams, they can afford reproducible and reliable information in regard to the trends of his thinking. These trends the psychiatrist may use in much the same manner as the internist does the chemical analyses of blood and urine.* Professors who make sweeping statements regarding the unscientific nature of psychiatry are guilty, as Dr. Eisenberg said, of a kind of negligence; they wouldn't dare speak in such a way regarding a comparable investigation of blood and urine.

Psychiatry, like any other discipline, is subject to criticism, but this is not a reason to exclude the discipline from the undergraduate medical curriculum. On the contrary, the very difficulties of this science and the contrast it affords with the

---

* An instance of the use of the content of a dream to guide psychotherapy is provided shortly by the patient who recounts his experience with migraine headaches.

exact sciences are reasons for its inclusion in the young doctor's educational program.

IS PSYCHOTHERAPY UNECONOMIC?

The third criticism of current psychotherapy is that it is inordinately time-consuming and uneconomic. This criticism is easily answered: it isn't always time-consuming, and when it is, it doesn't differ very much from physical modes of therapy, which thus far have not been bombarded with comparable criticism.

Those physicians who criticize psychotherapy because it takes too long are talking about long-term psychotherapy, or, in general, psychoanalysis. It is apparent that these physicians are unaware of the benefit many patients receive from a relatively few interviews with a psychiatrist. The following is an account written by a young lawyer of the benefit he received from some 50 psychiatric interviews.

What you said a few weeks ago about the psychological origins of disease put me in mind of my own experience with migraine headaches, and I think you may be interested to know my history. I cannot be precise about the time when I first started having headaches, but I think it was about 1943, when I was 14 or 15 years of age and went away to boarding school. The headaches were of the classic variety, beginning with a disturbance in my vision on one side (I cannot remember which one now), lasting perhaps 20 minutes or half an hour almost immediately followed by a nagging pain around the eye on the other side. I would sometimes wake up with a headache, or it would occur at any time during the day.

Medication did not relieve the pain. Since I was also debilitated by the occurrence, I often went to sleep if I could, and the pain was usually gone in an hour or two, although my head would throb if I exerted myself before the next day.

Several relatives on my father's side of the family had suffered from such headaches, my great aunt all her life in a more acute form, and my grandfather until he started taking cold baths in the morning, walking five miles to and from work every day, giving up coffee, chocolate—in short all the usual privations. It was, therefore, thought by some that my sufferings were hereditary and hopeless.

Since, however, we were acquainted with the world of Boston medicine, an extensive search for a cure was undertaken. I was examined thoroughly by a well-known internist; the studies included a metabolism test, an electrocardiogram and an electroencephalogram, I believe. I am sure I was also x-rayed. You can gauge the professional time involved. The results were all negative —as you doctors say—and so I proceeded to have my eyes examined, my teeth examined by my regular dentist, and finally my head examined by a neurologist, who said that the headaches were of the classic form, that he could not suggest a cure, but prescribed caffein pills to give me some relief. (I never understood why I should be helped by caffein pills if coffee were the cause of my difficulty.)

I received all of this attention prior to starting college in 1946, although I cannot give any precise dates. Since none of it seemed at all helpful, I concluded that I would have to live with my problem and expect a headache once or twice a month for the rest of my life. In fact, that *was* the pattern for the next ten years.

In the fall of 1957, I went to see a psychiatrist, not about the headaches—none of the eminent men or anyone else, for that matter, had suggested a psychological inquiry into the causes of that problem—but because I was anxious about something else. I laid my concern before the psychiatrist. In the course of our one interview, he discovered the headaches. He prescribed a Rorschach test, administered by a psychologist. When those results were in, he called me and advised me to see a therapist whom he recommended, not about the problem that had taken me to him, but about the headaches.

I saw the psychiatrist he recommended twice a week during the winter of 1957 and 1958. The night before one interview—I guess it was as early as the tenth we had had—I had a very vivid dream and woke up with a headache. Of course, that was the subject of our session the following afternoon, at which he linked the dream to the headache. The rest of the time I was seeing him I never had another headache. I think I have had only one thereafter, six months or so following the end of treatment. I don't believe that I saw him in total for more than 50 hours.

Countless such examples could be quoted.

Regarding long-term psychotherapy, it is true that the psychoanalytic process is time-consuming; many patients remain in psychoanalysis more than two years and some even four or five. Since the patient under analysis may have from 200 to 250 interviews with his psychiatrist each year, the minimum time involved in the psychoanalysis may be from 400 to 500 hours. (Each interview is usually 45 to 50 minutes; so the actual time spent by the patient is somewhat less, but the professional time of the doctor devoted to that patient is usually one hour.)

It is not surprising that the process of psychoanalysis should be so time-consuming. It is, in essence, a process of reeducation, for it is directed at helping the patient see that the habits of thought, which he fell into long ago, are now giving him trouble. It is very difficult for any of us to see why we think as we do about many subjects, and particularly about those important in orienting our way of life. If we are in trouble with our fellow beings, and this is the reason for which psychoanalysis is most often needed or recommended, it is particularly difficult to see where our thought processes are at loggerheads with society. The very approach to the difficulty leads us to shy away, as horses used to shy away in terror from locomotives or automobiles. The more troubled the patient, the more difficult the analytic process, and generally the more time-consuming—for both patient and psychiatrist.

The criticism of time is unfair from another point of view. I don't find these same critics complaining about the amount of professional time involved in many physical treatments. The average thyroidectomy, or gastrectomy or resection of the lung, requires 20 professional hours. This is doctor time and excludes all the time needed from nurses and orderlies, maintenance and other operating room personnel. In most hospital settings, the patient is admitted and worked up by the intern and resident. These same members of the house staff assist at the operation and care for the patient throughout the hospital convalescence. There is at least one anesthetist, sometimes an assistant anesthetist; and in general the anesthetist's time with the patient exceeds the actual operating time by one hour. In a university hospital setting, there are medical students who join in the care of the patient in collaboration with the house staff. Then, finally, there is the surgeon and perhaps his associate. As with the anesthetist, his time with the patient exceeds by at least an hour the time required for the operation. Many a patient with an emotional trouble may receive striking support from a psychiatrist in no more hours of psychotherapy.

A number of operations currently being performed across this country require far more than 20 professional hours of physician time. Recently, at the Massachusetts General Hospital, an older patient was rehabilitated after at least 240 professional hours had been devoted to him. This patient was a 67-

year-old man from another state, who had had an aneurysm of his abdominal aorta resected and replaced by a synthetic graft. The graft became infected, a small abscess formed, and a leak in the suture line resulted. A slow hemorrhage from the aorta occurred. At least 100 professional hours had been devoted to that man in the first hospital. At the Massachusetts General in the first week, a minimum of 140 physician hours were devoted to him. First came the studies by the roentgenologists. The leak in the suture line was not disclosed until the second study, and several days had passed before positive blood cultures were in. By the sixth day of hospitalization, when the diagnosis seemed assured, he was taken to the operating room, where $8\frac{1}{2}$ hours were spent before the old graft had been removed, the abscess identified and isolated, and a new graft placed in a new area providing for blood flow to both extremities and the organs below the diaphragm. I hear no criticism against such operations, and, indeed, there should be none. The people whose arteries plug off, or break, or rupture, or develop aneurysms are older people, but older people deserve care even if it is inordinately demanding of physicians' time and effort. The psychiatrist, in contrast to the surgeon, who cares for damaged, diseased blood vessels, deals more with younger people. It is the young who are accepted for psychoanalysis; they are best able to receive the benefit of reeducation and reorientation.

Other examples of diseases that require the time-consuming devotion of physicians are many. One with which I am familiar is the treatment of Graves' disease, by radioactive iodine. The treatment was first introduced in 1941, and became more generally available soon after World War II. It was heralded at first because of its simplicity and the minimum amount of time needed by the physician. Unfortunately, it has turned out that many of the patients eventually develop hypothyroidism, and they will obviously need the attention of a physician for the remainder of their lives. Before this complication of the therapy was recognized, many of the patients had become myxedematous, and it was difficult to bring them back smoothly to the normal level of thyroid function. The patient may be unaware of slipping into hypothyroidism. Even the family and friends may not notice the change because it occurs so slowly. Occasionally the use of thyroid therapy to bring the patient back to normal is accompanied by severe cardiac attacks and even death. At the present state of our knowledge, 40% of the patients treated with radioactive iodine have become hypothyroid, mild or severe, within the first ten years after the radiation therapy. It is possible that by reducing the initial dose of the irradiation, this undesirable result may be reduced—perhaps cut in half—but it will probably not be eliminated altogether, and since it is impossible to tell beforehand which patients will develop it, all patients who have had this therapy will have to be followed by their physicians. If the patient was aged 20 when receiving the therapy and lives to be aged 80, the number of professional hours that will be devoted to him over those 60 years adds up. Since Graves' disease will often yield to psychiatric treatment, some 60 hours of psychotherapy given to that patient at the age of 20 might well be regarded as time-saving in its life-long effect. The physician time, however, would be distributed differently.

FEES

Psychiatrists stand accused that they are overly concerned with their fees, and that their charges are inordinately high. Fees are a problem to many doctors. Some psychiatrists presumably have been rightly accused, but is it fair to level this charge against the psychiatrist alone? Other doctors have been equally guilty.

For the last three generations, surgeons have excused themselves for their high fees on the basis that the surgical training was prolonged, that the number of patients compared to all of the sick was small, and that the responsibility for the conduct of an operation was greater than that of most other medical treatments. Society has recognized the weight of these arguments by agreeing to pay high fees.

In much the same sense, the psychiatrist's training and education are prolonged, and the number of patients that he can treat in any one period is limited. His moral and ethical responsibility to the patient is high.

The psychiatrist is also criticized for arranging the fee before accepting the patient. But many other doctors do this. Many surgical patients prefer to know beforehand what the fee will be; therefore, many surgeons stipulate or discuss the fee for the proposed operation ahead of the fact. Indeed, the trend is towards prepayment or at least setting a fee ahead of time. Obstetricians set their fees, and several hospitals caring for people of moderate income scrupulously inform their patients ahead of time of the fee-for-service scale. The Baker Memorial division of the Massachusetts General Hospital in 1930 started informing each patient on entry of the surgical fee to be charged.

There is, further, a special reason that the psychiatrist discusses and settles the question of the fee beforehand. If the fee is of no consequence to the patient, he may take the interviews lightly. If, on the other hand, the fee is to some degree a burden to him, he is more certain to buckle down and work hard at his problem—and thereby shorten the length of treatment.

Group therapy has attempted to spread the effectiveness of a single psychiatrist. Although it has certain advantages, its limitations are also distinct, and it does not appear at the present to have advanced efficiency to any remarkable degree.

The whole matter of the cost of medical care and the fees charged by physicians needs reconsideration across the board. Perhaps the psychiatrist's fees are out of line and the economically less well off are not receiving their share of attention. Certainly surgical fees are disproportionately high, compared with the remuneration of many of our colleagues in internal medicine and its specialties. The entire medical profession needs to attend to these matters. The years of education need better support, and more attention should be given to the sharing of income in group endeavors. In the meantime, it is not fair or helpful to pick out the psychiatrists as a scapegoat.

LANGUAGE

The critics of psychiatry complain that psychiatry has developed a language of its own—a jargon often incomprehensible to most physicians. I think this criticism has some justification. A developing science may need to coin words of its own if there are no words available to provide the nearly exact meanings intended. In chemistry, for example, the English language had no single word to convey the meaning of such a substance as an enzyme; the name had to be manufactured. The entire industrial development is replete with the coinage of new words. To designate a particular wrench as a monkey wrench is to choose but one of countless examples. It is not only specific but telling.

The more precise and specific the meaning of a word, the better the communication between speaker and hearer, writer and reader. If all the words mean the same to both, the communication should be perfect. A word that permits confusion inserts uncertainty into the communication. Take for example, *id*. It is a word which in itself has endless meanings: thing. Everything is a thing. It is used by the psychiatrist, however, to indicate the basic instinctual drives. In a sense, it is the animal aspect of our behavior; it can mean sexual drive, protective instincts, appetites and craving. If what the psychiatrist wants to say is "craving," is it not much better to say that than to use "id"? And if the craving is sexual, is it not better to say that than leave the reader to infer that the craving was for chocolates? The one advantage to the word *id* is its brevity.

I can't help being reminded of Mark Twain's humorous account of the German language and *zug*.[26] He counted up some 28 separate usages for zug. It is obvious that when the German uses zug, the context tells him which particular meaning is intended; but I have never been quite sure when I read *id* just how much or how little I was to include in the meaning.

Recently there have been two charming and at the same time scathing articles on the use of language, Barbara Tuchman's "The Historian's Opportunity" in the *Saturday Review,* and Norman Cousin's editorial, "The Environment of Language" in the same magazine.[27, 28] Mrs. Tuchman had the following to say:

Historians can—though not all do—make themselves understood in every day English, the language in use from Chaucer to Churchill. Let us beware of the plight of our colleagues, the behavioral scientists, who by use of a proliferating jargon have painted themselves into a corner—or isolation ward—of unintelligibility. "They" know what they mean but no one else does. Psychologists and sociologists are the farthest gone in the disease and probably incurable. Their condition might be pitied if one did not suspect it was deliberate. Their retreat into the arcane is meant to set them apart from the great unlearned, to mark their possession of some unshared, unsharable expertise. No matter how illuminating their discoveries, if the behavioral scientists write only to be understood by one another, they must come to the end of the Mandarins.

Communication, after all, is what language was invented for. If history is to share its insights with a public in need of them, it must practice communication as an art, as Gibbon did, or Parkman.[27]

Norman Cousins speaks of studies in language going on at the Pro Deo University in Rome, which deal with "the dangerous misconceptions and prejudices that take root in language and undermine human values."

One of the more interesting papers being studied by the Pro Deo scholars is by Ossie Davis, the author and actor. Mr. Davis, a Negro, concluded on the basis of a detailed study of dictionaries and *Roget's Thesaurus* that the English language was his enemy. In Roget's, he counted 120 synonyms for "blackness," most of them with unpleasant connotations: blot, blotch, blight, smut, smudge, sully, begrime, soot, becloud, obscure, dingy, murky, threatening, frowning, foreboding, forbidden, sinister, baneful, dismal, evil, wicked, malignant, deadly, secretive, unclean, unwashed, foul, blacklist, black book, black-hearted, etc. Incorporated in the same listing were words such as Negro, nigger, and darky.

In the same *Roget's,* Mr. Davis found 134 synonyms for the word "white," almost all of them with favorable connotations: purity, cleanness, bright, shining, fair, blonde, stainless, chaste, unblemished, unsullied, innocent, honorable, upright, just, straightforward, genuine, trustworthy, honesty, etc. "White" as a racial designation was, of course, included in this tally of desirable terms.

. . . the word black in many African tongues has connotations of strength, certainty, recognizability, integrity, while white is associated with paleness, anemia, unnaturalness, deviousness, untrustworthiness.

Prejudice is not merely imparted or superimposed. It is metabolized in the bloodstream of society. What is needed is not so much a change in language as an awareness of the power of words to condition attitudes. . . .[28]

Medical people in general, and psychiatrists in particular, should be careful of their words. They must not misinterpret the language of the patient, and they should not compound trouble by themselves using words that may have double meanings.

AN END TO CRITICISM

I am deeply concerned by the criticism I still hear, in 1967, heaped upon psychiatrists and psychoanalysts by other members of the medical profession. The psychiatrists are striving to help sick people just as much as other clinical practitioners. They are just as conscientious and devoted. The psychiatrists' understanding of the problems they face may ultimately prove to have been misguided in much the same way and to the same degree that other theories in medicine have in the past so often proved misguided; no more, no less.

The psychiatrists deal with a field more complex and harder to grasp than any other of medicine. We others should be grateful to them for being brave—or foolhardy—enough to tackle the psychological problems of troubled people—grateful not carping. If, during the care of their patients, a patient should be found to harbor a somatic disease, for example Ca of the colon, we should not criticize—or gloat—unless we can be sure we have never overlooked anything in one of our patients, perhaps a carcinoma of the colon or stomach in a patient whose hernia we have just repaired. We should help, not hinder. The kinds of criticisms I hear have no place among scholars.

Psychiatrists are able to help us, if we will only listen. What is really important is that they are here and can help us. Carping criticism cuts us off from them at the very time that we should be seeking their help.

CHAPTER 5

To the Student

THE EXCITING PHASES in the development of medicine have been those of formative periods when uncertainty was rife and research rich. The discussions of the participants in this Study already described indicate the lack of agreement about almost everything, including definitions and what to do. About all the Study could agree upon was that behavioral science was important somehow in medicine. Behavioral science is thus in an evolutionary phase, and it will be in your professional lifetime that exciting developments will be taking place. You should have a part in them. How do you and your faculty go about this?

The evidence that the behavioral sciences can be important to the practice of medicine has been presented in Chapters 2 and 3. The role of the psychiatrist as a behavioral scientist, practitioner and teacher of medicine has been described in Chapter 4. There is nothing new in the evidence or descriptions. Leading medical educators have long been aware that psychiatry is essential and has needed its place in the medical curriculum. In 1934, Max Mason in his *Annual Report* to the Rockefeller Foundation said that the next big issue in medical education was behavioral science and psychiatry. Up until that time, the Foundation had been instrumental in starting full-time departments of the preclinical sciences and of internal medicine and surgery in a number of medical schools. Now they proposed to support psychiatry. In the succeeding years, with Rockefeller backing, full-time professors of psychiatry were appointed and departments of psychiatry developed in several medical schools. Next, the National Mental Health Act of 1946 introduced departments of psychiatry into all the remaining medical schools which had not had them. Still the desired objective is far from reached.

Before we go any further, let us understand that the exact sciences are essential underpinnings of modern medicine. Without mathematics, biophysics, biochemistry and physiology, medicine is as naught. But the exact or hard sciences, as we know them today, are not enough.

The practice of medicine is a combination of the science and art of medicine. The science is that part known with certainty; it is reproducible and predictable. Beyond the line of certainty lie concepts and theoretical projections into less well-charted areas, charted by experience alone. The art of medicine takes in the concepts and experience in these little charted areas. Obviously this definition of the art is not that of the plastic surgeon used in reshaping a scarred face; it is an art which stems from intuition, an art guided by experience. Someone once said that the art of living is the ability to make the right decision on inadequate evidence. The art of medicine is also the ability to make the right decision on inadequate evidence.

If this definition of the practice of medicine is accepted, then there are several matters of consequence in regard to the art—of consequence not alone to its use in practice but to its role in the progress of medicine and to its teaching. There will always be an art to the practice of good medicine, because it can be assumed that there will always be a limit to what is known with certainty, and beyond that limit the physician will have to grope his way. Try he must as best he can, for he has no alternative. He may not send the patient home to return a year hence when more might be known about the patient's disease. The physician who limits his medicine to what he knows to be truly established is a hobbled man indeed.

The second matter of consequence to the art of medicine is its double significance in relation to the use of behavioral science. The hard sciences of medicine have given us much to practice with, and the need for the art is less acute and less demanding. Concepts and projections into the unknown have a sturdy foundation; there is less risk to the art. Not so when it comes to the areas involving behavioral science. So much less is certain. The doctor treating patients with emotional difficulties is by necessity forced into using more theory and making more assumptions than when he is dealing with many of the somatic troubles. He is thus doubly dependent on his judgment, his experience, his art.

The third matter of consequence is that there is an art to the progress of medicine itself, an art as important as that of the practice. Every progressive science has its art—the intuition that leads the investigator to the next step in his experiments. It is the art essential to the research which is in turn essential to sound progress.

Finally, if our definition of practice holds, then it is the art of medicine, not the science, that is difficult—difficult to practice but above all difficult to teach. That it is relatively easy to teach the science of medicine should not be surprising. In this modern world, we have every facility for the teaching of science, particularly the hard sciences—books, movies, and laboratories galore, with materials and models to illustrate every conceivable point.

Not so the art. By definition, we are not sure of our premises. We move on the basis of assumptions, and these must be tested at every turn. We have no fixed laboratory. Every human being is different. We have to devise our materials and models as we go. Progress is slow and uncertain, and we are dependent upon experience.

Without experience, there can be no reliable intuition—no reliable art. Unfortunately, experience is the biggest hurdle of education. No generation has succeeded in teaching it to the next in a short time. Precept may be a guide and the teacher may help by suggesting and criticizing, but experience can come only with living. Opportunity, time, and an unprejudiced spirit of inquiry—these are requisites.

Experience: Laboratory of the Art

What we seek is experience, and the laboratory we need we may call the laboratory of the Art of Medicine. It must be a laboratory in which we can make observations, gather data, look for things which are comparable and which may be wound into concept or theory we can use in practice. An element of research will always be involved in the laboratory of the art, and

the effort at research distinguishes between limited and expand-
ing good medicine. There is always more before us than we can
see.

Second, it is essential to our eventual practice of the art that
we acquire the habit of striving to see more. We must bear in
mind that students and practitioners of medicine tend to relax
within the boundaries of the science of medicine. They are
tempted to stick to what is known, because then they are on
solid ground, as solid as the scientific evidence or data afford.

Those learning or practicing the art·of medicine are on more
shaky grounds. The amount of reproducible data is limited and
the need for checking at every point more urgent. This striving
demands of us constant effort, a will to see, and a spirit of
unprejudiced inquiry. Let us see what Dr. Aring has to say
about experience.

The Uses of Personal Experience

First, I want to commune with our junior partners, the students
of medicine. They are always my first concern. I find them needing
the assurance that all of their experience bears on practice. Everything we have met can be put to use for the benefit of patients; it is
all grist for this mill. Personal experience, before medical school
and outside it, is useful in caring for patients. Medical faculties
have a studied way of ignoring the particular experiences and tal-
ents of students, as though they didn't matter. This strikes me as a
part of the decline of all arts in an era of scientism. Since Descartes,
we have fostered a mechanistic and laboratory orientation of medicine, the pure and simple scientific approach. A sterile environment
allows vulnerability, and lack of exposure to some of the transac-
tions that make for vigorous humanity is hobbling. In medicine, I
consider it a pedagogic duty to direct the development of any talent
into competence. It isn't as though medical students were ignorant;
rather they are clumsy, about as clumsy as we were when we were
junior. A natural concern by seniors for the ideas, abilities, and
ideals of their juniors is useful. When something of importance to a
developing personality is ignored or is not worked through, as the
psychiatrists say, it becomes hedged round with derivatives not particularly constructive.

I urge our junior partners to bring to practice all their experience. It is useful and will fit somewhere.[5]

What are the experiences Dr. Aring is talking about? They
are of many sorts—contacts with animals, things observed and

felt about people—family, teachers, friends, yourselves and what you have read.

FARM LIFE: AN EARLY LABORATORY

Lucky is he who has been brought up on a farm, for he will have had valuable experience watching how animals behave. He will know what the shelter and safety of the barn mean to the horse or cow. Should the barn catch on fire and the horse be aware of danger, it is almost impossible to dislodge him, and he will be consumed in the fire. That boy or girl will have learnt the meaning of horse sense—how fundamental, but how limited. For him it is less necessary to study the life of the baboon. But for a student brought up in an urban environment who has never had a dog or watched a dog dreaming, chasing rabbits, it will be important to gain an intimate acquaintance with animals.

The dog, the horse, and the cow are not human beings. Their behavior, however, in many respects gives a good view of the underlying animal instincts of the human being. Not only do animals and human beings resemble each other in such instinctual drives as defense, sex, and withdrawal in the face of threat or excessive anxiety, but the human being also shares with the animal changes in feeling of well-being with the season and the climate. The increment and decrement of daylight, which determine the egg-laying and molting season of the domestic hen and the spawning of the trout, also influence the intensity of such common conditions as exophthalmic goiter. The poets, since time immemorial, have recognized the effect of the seasons —for instance, the effect of the spring on our sense of well-being.

THE LABORATORY OF EVERYDAY HUMAN CONTACT

As I have said, observation of animals may help in our understanding of the fundamental animal-like instincts of the human being, but there is a strict limitation to the understanding of human behavior that animals give us. The vagaries and foibles of our thinking, though influenced by our mammalian instincts, are controlled and tangled in our higher centers. It is only by observing people and examining our own thinking that we can come to understand the human being in health and disease.

Most of us, in a rudimentary way, have given thought to the problem of understanding people. For many it will have been a part of family life. Others will have studied psychology and the social sciences in college, and will have been thrown with people of unusual human understanding. Others may have come from families in which discussions of personalities were avoided for fear of unkind criticisms. For them, the start may be more difficult, but so much more important. All of us have traditional psychological approaches which we must look into carefully in order to understand, if we can, our reticences and prejudices.

In medical school, understanding people should be a concerted project not left to chance. We should start with ourselves and our own lives rather than with patients; much can be learned by looking back at our families and upbringing. Next come our teachers. What have they taught us about people? What can we learn by looking at their approaches to people? How did it happen that we became interested in medicine? Is it possible to be interested in medicine but not in people; how could this be? Of the medical faculty, some are interested in people and others not. Is their interest divided according to discipline, or to their occupation, their family background, or chance?

That a man is a chemist does not mean he is insensitive to human values. By the same token, it does not follow that clinicians who are dealing daily with patients are sensitive and aware of the emotional troubles of their patients. Sensitivity to human qualities of people is not associated with, or excluded by, any one discipline. Theoretically, interest and competence in dealing with human values might be less likely among scholars especially concerned with those aspects of hard science basic to medicine, and should be in greater abundance among those who are supposedly dealing with the human aspects of the patient. The division does not turn out to be like that. To me, the widespread prescription of tranquilizers by physicians and surgeons, the number of doctors who count on this short-cut temporary approach to emotional complaints, is a firm indication of the truth of this assertion.

Much can be accomplished by talking with one's peers. In any group, there will be people of different points of view and different reactions; comparing them may be a good way to start.

There are some inherent dangers, however, in probing too far in an amateurish way. While looking into our own recesses and those of others, we may form strong likes and dislikes. Listening to others and then recounting our own experiences can be heady stuff. Like wine, it can lead us down unhealthful paths. The present trends to LSD and marijuana are, perhaps, examples of an interested search into the inner mind of self and others. Alcohol used to suffice and perhaps was a safer approach. But even the use of alcohol as a means of putting aside our inhibitions and opening our hearts can have dire consequences to personal behavior and to subsequent professional competence and reputation.

I am suggesting that the sharing of confidences by amateurs and without the guidance of more mature and experienced persons may lead to unwise dislikes or attachments. There is also an occasional danger from the unskilled release of buried materials. Yet it is essential to come to understand our peers and above all ourselves. How can we bring this about?

It is almost impossible, no matter how well meaning we are, to examine our own processes of thought without the help of others. Rare is the human being who can see through his own foibles, his own repressions. It is true that after learning to see through our own restraints we can go quite a distance in realizing the reasons we do things, but most of us have needed the guiding hand of an experienced observer of the mind.

It should be the responsibility of the faculty to make available to students as individuals, or to groups of students, competent tutors who will help in these approaches to the understanding of personality. Faculties are made up of human beings, however, and teachers have their own reticences. They may hesitate to offer their services formally. In fact, often the most understanding people are the least aggressive and talkative, and they have to be sought out. They are to be found, however, always ready to talk, since anybody who is understanding of himself enjoys the presence of others, no matter what the age difference.

Two more points about the study of oneself in the laboratory of personal experience. First, pay attention to your dreams. If you don't realize you have them, watch out for them; they are there. Dreams are the most direct line to what is going on in our minds just under cover of our conscious thoughts. Certainly they are a most important line to our automatic pilot. Second, read widely. There is no need to be bored. Good novels and good biography offer sensitive views of people.

THE DEVELOPMENT OF EXPERIENCE IN THE CARE OF THE PATIENT

All that I have written has been said, in one way or another, by the participants of the Study. There were several practical suggestions as to how the experiments could be carried out in the laboratory of experience: I refer you particularly to the illustrations of Dr. Leaf's and Dr. Solnit's committee in Appendix D. When it came to developing an experience with the patient, opinions differed somewhat. Dr. Eisenberg felt that we as teachers are overly concerned about the harm that students can do to patients, even when the students are adequately supervised.* He advised bringing students in contact with patients as early as possible. Others hesitated to have inexperienced students question patients about their emotional problems. They felt that the student should have experience in understanding himself, and in delving into the thinking of well-balanced normal individuals, before probing into the lives of the sick. This difference in point of view applies to the physical sciences of disease and the physical examination of the patient. Some teachers of medicine advise that students plunge right into pathology, both in its theoretical aspect and as it is encountered in the living patient. Others, and this is the traditional point of view, hold that the student should understand, first, normal anatomy in all its intricacies and, next, physiology, biophysics and biochemistry. When these are known, then he should study the disordered pathology of disease as it appears in the patient.

---

* At several points in the Study, the educational value of mistakes was discussed. The traditional point of view is to hold the student at arm's length from the patient until he knows enough not to make a mistake. Dr. Eisenberg thought the student should be encouraged to try himself out earlier.

Certainly I have learned a lot from my mistakes, but I don't think I would recommend making mistakes as an approach to learning. Some of mine were bad boners. A trouble with mistakes is that they are by no means always recognized. When things go well, there may still be a mistake or even several, but because of the success they are glossed over.

There is no one formula to an education, and much will depend on you and your teachers. In recent years in the pre-clinical sciences, there has been a trend to bring you in contact early with disease, and by this approach help you to understand the meaning for the studies of anatomy and physiology. Likewise, in relation to the behavioral aspect of medicine, it will be wise if your faculty introduces you to patients early. Thus you will come to see the need to study yourself, your own thinking, and that of other normal individuals.

Regarding the study of the patient, I recommend particularly the report of Drs. Solnit and Provence—Appendix D. In it there are many helpful suggestions as to how to go about it.

In your contact with the patient and the subsequent writing of the record, you may find it helpful to consider those things you note about the patient's behavior under Behavior Examination, a designation separate from History and Physical Examination. During World War II, Dr. Stanley Cobb, Dr. Jacob Finesinger, and other members of the Department of Psychiatry at Harvard advised the Curriculum Committee to reorganize the traditional pattern of the patient record. The record at that time consisted of three parts, History, Physical Examination, and Diagnostic Impression. The only words regarding the patient's emotional attitudes and behavior were included under Mental Status—the last of 16 items of the Physical Examination. Mental Status was accorded no greater weight than Rectum or Extremities, two others of the 16 items. They called the faculty's attention to the advisability of observing the patient's behavior both while taking the history and carrying out the physical examination; much could be learned of importance to the diagnosis. To impress those matters on the student and the young doctor, they suggested adding the Behavior Examination as a fourth part of the official record form. Besides, there was no proper place to record the patient's reactions in the History or the behavior under Mental Status. With increasing knowledge, more room was needed to include the behavioral observations important to the diagnosis.

At the time this fourth item of the hospital work-up was introduced in 1948, the faculty was unable to appreciate its importance. Except for a transient period it has hardly ever been used. This is unfortunate, for it has so much to offer.

BEWARE OF THE CHANGE IN ATTITUDE

Something happens to many students during the under-graduate medical years, or just afterwards in the internship. The attitude toward patients may shift from one of interest in them as human beings with feelings like their own, to a cold-roast attitude in which all that is important is the hard science aspect of diagnosis and treatment. The human interest gets ground out. Anxieties and such complaints as headaches with no organic lesions to be found become "imaginary," not real like a "real tumor" or a "real pain."

This change in attitude is highly undesirable. Serious misconceptions result, and patient care suffers. There is nothing imaginary about a headache. To the patient it is real. The patient is not fibbing or trying to mislead the doctor; he is only reporting and asking for help. So it is also with other so-called "imaginary complaints."

There are many reasons behind this change in attitude, and you should be sure that you are aware of them so that you too will not shift. Dr. Bondy has summarized the factors admirably in Appendix C. Of especial note is the following:

Dr. Bondy: A number of the factors that lead to these changes can be suggested. First, the need of the student to develop a *protective carapace* so that he can tolerate the unpleasant experiences of the clinic. At some time in his professional training, each student must learn to handle the emotional disturbance caused by his patients' suffering without allowing it to overwhelm him. He will often be confronted with tragedy that he cannot alleviate or with pain that he must tolerate or even himself inflict. If he allows himself to be too upset by these necessary aspects of the healing art, he will not be able to function effectively. One of his earliest tasks in the clinic will be to apply dispassionate, intellectual processes to studying disturbing, painful or even disgusting aspects of human suffering. Unless he can learn this dispassionate attitude, he will never be an effective physician. On the other hand, somewhere along the line he must develop a balanced attitude which does not exclude a recognition of the social, behavioral and psychiatric factors which make the patient a person rather than simply an intellectual problem in disordered physiology. The development of this *balance* takes time and experience. The first step usually represents an *overshoot* in the direction of "toughness" and cynicism.

Don't stop with this one paragraph. Read all that Dr. Bondy has to say.

Perhaps another reason, not specifically alluded to by Dr. Bondy, impels some students to the cold side of medical practice, and this is the seductive nature of human intimacy. I have already alluded to this problem of intimacy under the dangers of probing into personalities and the need for help from the faculty. Biologically, the problem seems to me to have a simple origin. No one of us is complete, male or female. Alone, each of us is inadequate. We need the complement of another person, or at least an animal such as a dog. This need for company is deep-rooted in us, and the exchange of inner personal thoughts and of emotional troubles between two human beings can be seductive.

It is something of this basic biologic need for another person that may lead us into trouble as physicians. For example, the neurotic, hysterical woman enthralls the unwary doctor, and out of this enthrallment come unnecessary operations, unnecessary drugs, prolonged hospitalizations, and unnecessary visits to the doctor. Because of the fear of being bitten, some young physicians shy away from human contacts. Perhaps, down underneath, they want the contact too much themselves.

To offset this pitfall, the psychiatrist stresses the distinction between sympathy and empathy. The doctor is to be wary of sympathy, for it may lead him into becoming involved, into being carried away emotionally. Empathy, however, he should have in order to understand his patient.* It is a neat balance.

BEWARE THE SYSTEM OF STUDIES

There are grave disadvantages to the examination and marking systems current in most American medical schools. The student isn't allowed to examine the subject on his own. The pace of the medical curriculum is demanding and leaves no spare time; the character of the examinations demands that the student follow the program set by the teacher. Both are stultifying, for they cut the student off from taking the initiative for what he is to learn. Another disadvantage of the current marking system is that too many of us hesitate to try out an idea before our peers and certainly before our teachers if we think it may be

---

* Empathy is defined as the imaginative projection of one's own consciousness into another being, and so fully understanding the object of contemplation (combination of The Oxford and Webster's Dictionaries).

wrong. Marks count for too much and all know this. In a competitive world such as medicine who is going to discount his possibility for a good internship by saying something that may be interpreted as being a bit foolish? Obviously, I don't suggest saying foolish things, but the student should feel sufficiently free in his relationship with instructors and fellow students to explore ideas to the fullest and determine their limitations.

COMPUTER MEDICINE

At this moment, a strong and special reason looms for students of medicine to concern themselves early with behavioral science both in understanding themselves and the emotional make-up of others. That reason is the approach of computer medicine. It can be seen now that several aspects of medicine can be expedited by computers. Some of the diagnostic work-up, particularly that related to the hard measurements of diagnosis, can be called for, arranged, dictated, enumerated, transcribed entirely through computers and without the interference of physician or physician assistant. Not so the behavioral aspect of the patient and his care. We just don't know enough at the present time to program a computer with the emotional aspects of the patient. This is where the art of medicine ranges into scarcely defined areas. A physician, an educated sensitive physician, is needed. Perhaps as our understanding of patient behavior becomes more explicit, then aspects could be fed through a properly programed computer, but this seems to be far away. First, we must educate the physician.

The rising costs of medical care are driving us toward computer medicine. Concern over costs will also affect the character of care in other ways. This concern is already leading us to try to extend the doctor's effectiveness, to streamline his efficiency by measures other than computers. This will mean inevitably that the doctor will spend less time with each patient. The participants of this Study, indeed all good doctors, know that time with the patient is essential if emotional troubles of the patient are to come to the surface. A common complaint of patients already is that the doctor has so little time.*

* The following example of time spent with patients is a tragicomedy. A busy obstetrician of my acquaintance makes his morning rounds be-

Computer medicine may have a greater usefulness in such narrow areas of practice as battle casualties or military medicine in general. But in civilian medicine the problems are so multitudinous and various that there is rarely a special focus, and the apparent focus may be misleading or altogether wrong. No special form can be concocted for the patient to fill out that can conceivably cover all the possibilities or vagaries of human nature.

To the Next Generation

To return to behavioral science, the participants of this Study have the impression that there has been a long delay in the acceptance of behavioral science as an essential discipline of medicine and medical education. It took many years for chemistry to be acknowledged as important to the understanding of biology. Yet, as the science of biochemistry emerged, it was accepted by medicine without frustration or antagonism. Indeed, it has been greeted with enthusiasm. Everybody in medicine is wild about chemistry. Why the difference between the acceptance of chemistry and behavioral science?

There are many thoughts about this long delay and all are especially relevant to you, the students. Nothing is going to happen if you don't do it. The discussion among the participants of the Conference showed how faculties are stalled. Faculties are made up of successful and busy men. Their ideas have in large part crystallized during the most productive phases of their lives. Perhaps it is asking more than is reasonable to expect them under the heavy burden of academic life to stop and give adequate thought. In addition to this, the very thoughts needed are a bit perilous, anxiety-producing. But what a man of sixty cannot do, you in your formative years should be able to do. You are the cambium layer of the academic tree.

---

tween 6 and 7 A.M. He boasts that this early visiting hour saves him time. At that early hour in the morning, his patients have not had the time to wash their faces and put on their make-ups. They feel awkward when he visits, and avoid keeping him longer in the room. He escapes, therefore, without having answered their questions. This seems a harsh treatment where so many mothers—and most of them are young—must have many questions on their minds.

CHAPTER 6

To the Faculty

To THE FACULTY is addressed to those of you who are still with us. The others have stopped reading long ago. But you have kept an open mind on these matters and must be interested.

The participants felt that the solution of the problems lies in education. The behavioral sciences constitute a substantial group of scientific disciplines important to the practice of medicine. There was no doubt about this, though there was no unanimity regarding the specific applications. Medicine in the United States is far from convinced. Important islands of understanding have integrated behavioral science, including psychiatry, into teaching and practice, and have accepted the psychiatrist as a full partner in clinical medicine. But these islands are still few, despite 40 years of persistent effort.

Somehow, the educational process has failed to establish behavioral science as one of the doctor's useful tools. Students, graduates, and faculty are not so impressed with behavioral science as they are with the exact sciences. The psychiatrist continues to be shunned. This is our problem. What is wrong now and what do we need to do? First, let's look at what we are doing now.

American medical schools have made a variety of efforts to teach behavioral science, and psychiatry in particular. A number of schools have brief introductory courses to psychiatry in the first two years, running concurrently with the preclinical science courses. These are followed by formal courses in psychiatry in the clinical years. The introductory courses have been organized to catch the student's attention. They have been difficult to teach, and are more or less successful according to the intent and collaboration of the faculty as a whole. At Harvard, where psychiatry has had hard sledding, the introductory course was camouflaged under the name "Growth and Development"; embryology nominally is given equal value with the whole of behavioral science. Courses such as these have not proved automatically or continuously successful.

The participants discussed at length the various ways the medical schools are currently meeting this educational problem. Suggestions for improvement were diverse.

First, the place to teach behavioral science, many thought, is in college. Dr. Hunt and the anthropologists pointed out that numerous colleges have excellent departments of sociology, psychology, and cultural anthropology, where the prospective student can obtain a broad base of understanding. Medical schools should encourage prospective students to study in these departments and should alter their admission requirements in this direction.

Closely allied to the problem of teaching behavioral science in college is the question of the medical school's relations with the college of arts and sciences, and indeed with the whole university. Dr. Wedgwood and several others felt that the problems could best be met by bringing the medical school back into the university.

Dr. Wedgwood: The reason that we are really here is that the Endicott House Conference in part failed. It is quite apparent that there is an obvious territorial battle going on, with multiple cross-fires. The medical student is caught between them. What we have got to discuss . . . is not the place of the behavioral sciences in the medical school, but the place of a medical school in a university, and also the place of the medical school in society. To my mind, what you come down to is a good and solid discussion of what I term "the open university."

Dr. Zacharias: Maybe I am the only one here who has never worked in a medical school, and maybe for that reason I believe that the arbitrary separation of the medical school from the university and the college is a national scandal.

No matter how well behavioral science is taught in the preparatory college years, it was clear that the teaching of behavioral science and psychiatry in particular must be carried on throughout the formal undergraduate medical curriculum. Some of the participants felt that we should follow the example of the University of Kentucky, and set up within the medical faculty a separate department of behavioral science. Dr. Straus told us how he has learned to work with the clinical departments, bringing the student, intern and resident in touch with the social and behavioral aspects of their patients. We were impressed with his collaborative approach. The recommendation of a separate department was discussed at length by Dr. Beck's committee and appears in summary form in his report; see Appendix B.

Several of the participants would hesitate to found a separate department of behavioral science comparable to those of physiology and biochemistry. Dr. Freedman in particular felt that this would be unwise. The following discussion took place one afternoon:

Dr. Kety: If the behavioral sciences are as important as some of us think they are, why shouldn't they be departments of a medical school instead of adventitious appendages to some other department?

Dr. Zacharias: I would agree with you on that. Now is the time for departments of behavioral sciences to be independent.

Dr. Freedman: Strategically, politically and from an educational point of view, it probably isn't timely in most places to have departments of behavioral science. We have to watch out especially for physicians who chuck the responsibilities to someone else. It is like the old problem of a psychiatric referral. The physician names something and somebody else now will take over the responsibility for this area. Well, this depends on who the physician is and how he develops. . . .

Dr. Kety: It is unfortunate that the very important question of departmental structure is raised at a time when it may confuse the issue of the importance of the behavioral sciences. It may be wise to alter the organization of medical schools, and do away with traditional departments, although I am still to be convinced, but that does not affect the question of whether or not the behavioral sciences are an appropriate part of the medical curriculum and to be treated as such or merely a subdivision of one of the clinical specialties. It was not too long ago that biochemistry was fighting for recognition as a discipline in the medical faculty.

As an alternative to setting up a separate department of behavioral science within the medical school, Dr. Bond suggested that young men and women from the clinical departments be encouraged to join in the research of departments of behavioral science for a year or two, then to return to their own department.

Dr. Bond: On what to do about behavioral sciences in schools of medicine, it seems to me there is an extremely clear way. The best way is to have a professor of medicine who says, "I have to do something about this social science, or whatever it is you want to call it. I am going to get a bright young guy whom I trust. I trust him because I brought him up myself, so I know he is well trained, and this man has certain competences that I have tested. He has an interest in this area. I am going to send him over to some behavioral science or some social science department for a couple of years. Then he is going to come back because if I send him over, he will be a fine screen through which can pass a whole lot of stuff, a lot of it irrelevant; but this man, because he knows to what he wants to apply it, will know what to filter. I will bring him back, and he will apply it in my department." This is perhaps not the way it should end up, but I am convinced that this is the way it should start, because if somebody wants a little biochemistry even in pediatrics, what do you do? You get a bright young guy that you think has some promise. You send him over to a chemist you think has some knowledge. He doesn't come back if you don't make him come back or want him to come back. It may develop finally into something else. . . . But if you bring a lot of homeless characters from other fields such as the social sciences and dump them in a medical center and think they are going to do something, they're not. They're not going to do anything. You have to provide a home, and you don't send your dumbest resident over there either. You send your best resident. You say, go over there and see if you can make any sense out of this and bring it back and see if it has any application to medicine.

Dr. Wedgwood: The problem here is that each department will become a whole medical school in itself. Each medical school will become a university.

Dr. Bond: I don't believe it. I am saying this is the way you start.

Dr. Wedgwood: The problem of size relates to the problem of when does a medical school cease attempting to incorporate within its own structure the entire universe of human biology and human experience. When does a medical school open its doors to its students so they can go out into the university in which, by and large, the universes of human biology and human experience are represented as available disciplines.

Dr. Bond: This business of how big does anything get? I think Jerrold Zacharias has a sneaking answer to questions like that; it is a matter of taste. You want enough but not too many. You can't be too small, because your own knowledge is too limited and you have to have another person who is fairly smart whom you can at least fight with if you can't do anything else with him. You have to have a little interaction because he will ask you some questions you never thought of. I think that the major thing in this whole business is not getting answers out of it but at least figuring out what the major questions are. You don't get a lot of a distance with answers until you have some sort of question. The trouble with our questions at the moment is that they are the wrong size for our answers. . . .

All I am trying to say to these people is that they have got to have an entrance marked "Welcome." You take a sociologist or somebody, and you throw him into Bellevue Hospital and say: Swim, and nobody knows who he is. Somebody goes to talk to a patient; somebody gets mad at him. You have got to give the guy some protection when he is starting new in a new place. You can't smother him. You have got to give him a certain freedom to grow, but you have got to protect him. A lot of sociologists cannot be relevant at first. Many are quite irritated with the profession of medicine and, when plunged into an unfamiliar place, express it. Many wish they had become physicians themselves. The advantage of having a young physician get training in behavioral sciences and return is that he can be a sensitive bridge between the physicians and the social or behavioral scientists. He will be a fine entrance for all these other guys. He can talk to them, and he will take them around and introduce them to people. He will say it is okay for them to come on the wards; it is okay if they sit in the OPD. Let them make all the observations they want. You throw them in and you kill them. I have seen them die.

Dr. Hunt: What Doug has suggested is extremely important and a highly practical way of screening out and thinking up what is relevant. These behavioral sciences, you know, are departments of the graduate school. They have their own agenda; these fields have organization. They are not worried about the practice of medicine. They are developing their own fields. Of course, when they are brought in cold, they are going to be irrelevant because their stuff isn't about the practice of medicine; it is about sociology; it is about psychology; it isn't about how to cure people.

Dr. Bond: One other thing too. It is marvelous to be able to say, "This guy has such a commitment to this field that he was willing to send me away for a couple of years and then guarantee me a house when I return." That commitment says we want this stuff in here. That is very important, the commitment. This isn't done by words; it is done by action. There is nothing that speaks as loud as that action.

Dr. Quarton approached the problem of teaching behavioral science from three different angles: teacher training, innovation in teaching, and new three-year experimental medical schools.

Dr. Quarton: A lot of our teachers are really not motivated to teach, and some who are motivated don't know how. It is conceivable that the way to learn behavioral sciences is to approach it through work with teachers and as a separate task, through innovations in teaching. How to get teachers to make more of a contribution and innovation in teaching are not the same issue. Each deserves special consideration.

Radical innovations should be tried somewhere. Trial and error should be a better way of finding out what works than to sit in a committee and guess what works or use reasoning of one kind or another based on our own particular experience and training. None of the methods for teaching many of the things I have been trained for in medical school work terribly well and the only way to find out is to try experiments. I do regard the Western Reserve as a halfway successful experiment, which is an awfully good result, the best we have; but it has failed a little bit too and I would like to know why and how it doesn't work as well as people would like it to work. This belongs in a discussion of innovations. Instead of worrying about whether we should teach sociology to medical students, we should ask ourselves: Is there a place somewhere where a medical school could be set up to try some new things?

It should be possible to invent some new institutions that are not quite like existing medical schools but could teach very good methods. I would like to propose a special kind of medical school that would be cheaper than the regular medical school, that would be set up to do innovated teaching, have separate budgets and separate funds and would in a way be grafted onto existing medical schools to ensure the maintenance of standards. Such a school would not hurt the students. You could do what you really need to do, try different things out with a half-life to the program. What is wrong now is that when a program is started, professors are appointed for a life-time and they are frozen to defending what they have always done. If you ask them if they're doing a good job, they have to say yes because their whole career depends on this factor. We need ways to develop an institution in which we can try teaching behavioral science in a three-year span and then the whole experiment is over. If there is any value to it at all, it will be judged by what people will have seen and what the students say.

Dr. Child: We have tried at Michigan to start a new parallel school, but the plans have finally hit a snag. We were going to have a university of medicine, and it got along until some people felt that because it was so interesting this would be unfair to the students. Inevitably, the new plan would succeed and you couldn't have some students being shown preferential treatment. The whole plan fell down. The last thing they threw at it was that somebody said there would be no money.

Dr. Zacharias: It is important to emphasize this discussion because one of the things that shocked me after the Endicott House Study was to learn that the new medical schools forming were going to be just as conservative or reactionary as the ones that already had heads of anatomy departments.

Maybe we could recruit a group of interested faculty to plan and get something started.

Dr. Quarton: I don't think anyone here has the monopoly of knowledge on what the innovations should be. Almost everyone here should be able to come up with some plan. If there are some people who are more interested in it, that might be a better way of getting a report written that would stress the values of innovation in science teaching. I think it is true with teacher training; in other words, there are rather radical suggestions that one can make about how medical educators can become more sophisticated as teachers without going to an Education school. I happen to think that this whole group has something to say to this rather than assigning it to a small group of us who happen to be interested in it. I am a great believer in not talking about two things at once, and this is what we tend to do over and over again, going around in circles.

I am careful not to call innovation an experiment. I don't think you can set up controlled experiments. On the other hand, something can be learned by trying things not ordinarily tried.

A primary reason that it is difficult to get medicine to pay attention to behavioral science and psychiatry is that each of us thinks he knows about human behavior and what constitutes good and bad psychiatry. A big part of growing up is learning what makes people tick. We instinctively judge everybody we meet, and we doctors come to think of ourselves as authorities, each our own psychiatrist. This is something akin to considering ourselves authorities on politics; we know what is right and wrong, good and bad in politics, and we seldom change our political persuasion.

But politics and psychiatry are different. Part of democracy is voting and so we must make up our minds, have an opinion even though a superficial one. Not so psychiatry. There is a large and growing body of knowledge and a know-how in the care of the disturbed which few of us possess. Few of us are authorities. Unfortunately, it is only the unusual doctor who realizes the limitations of his knowledge, and, as in politics, it is the rare doctor who changes his point of view.

As a consequence of the feeling that each of us is an authority in psychiatry, we are faced with the ridiculous situation of doctors being wary about making any statement regarding such a hard science area as an enzyme system, about which they know little, yet willing in the next breath to make sweeping dogmatic statements about psychiatry, a field so complicated and so difficult to understand.

A second obstacle to the teaching of psychiatry lies in the very special material involved. Mental disturbances and psychiatry are full of upsetting thoughts, and we instinctively close our minds to them. We have all been well trained in how to do this in our infancy and childhood, and we are not quick to learn new habits any more than an old dog learns new tricks. So it is in a Study like ours that it is difficult to listen to others and change our minds. To expect established, effective teachers to go against the grain of habits of thinking dating from early childhood is too much to ask in two weeks of meetings. A far longer time is needed.

These two attitudes together mean that in general medical faculties are opposed to psychiatry. Where this situation exists, the efforts of an enlightened few can be undercut by a resistant majority. It is obviously too much to expect an established faculty to change its corporate point of view.* The teachers of medicine are appointed to medical faculties because they are effective people in their own fields, and are not impressed by the relevance of new knowledge in other fields.

There are also some not-so-subtle ways of defeating a movement or such a project as introducing behavioral science into the teaching program. Dr. Snyder pointed out that an overt principle of the faculty can be nullified covertly by examinations. The engineering faculty at MIT asks the students to be creative and imaginative in their studies, but forces them in the opposite direction by a rigid and demanding examination system.

* It was for this reason that Professor Zacharias suggested that this account of the Study of Behavioral Science be addressed to the students.

Concerning the question of organizing a separate department of behavioral science in the medical school, Dr. Freedman's reservation is cogent. The "chucking of responsibility" to someone else is an old and undesirable phenomenon in the practice of medicine. Surgeons in particular are to be found shrugging off responsibilities onto the shoulders of internist colleagues. This is not good; the patient too often gets lost between surgeon and internist. I refer to such matters as the fluid and electrolyte balance and chemotherapy of patients before and after operation.

Additional points against a separate department of behavioral science are the tendencies for all departmental walls to diminish communication and for departments to become fiefdoms, the property of the professor, to be zealously guarded against intrusions and inroads. Professor Whittemore and Mr. Katan, in their cogent and witty "Critical Appraisal and Exhortation from Two Laymen" (Appendix G), suggest that adding a department of behavioral science is "letting the science in without a fuss," brushing the dust under the rug, so to speak.

Enlightening comparisons are found in the experiences of insinuating into medicine both biochemistry and preventive medicine. Clinicians at first had a difficult time understanding the need for chemistry in their practice. Biochemistry had not arrived as a separate discipline in the college faculties of chemistry, and historically it appears that much was accomplished by instituting a department of biochemistry to teach in the first year of medical school. In the first generation following this development, biochemistry became firmly implanted in the practice of medicine.

In contrast, preventive medicine has not fared so well. Separate departments of preventive medicine have existed for at least two generations, and they have been run by splendid men; but they have had surprisingly little influence on the tenor of medical practice. Some think that this is because American medicine is rooted in the fee-for-service system, but it is more than that. Even in the prepayment clinic, where there is no fee-for-service, the doctor's fascination is with disease. It has been an uphill battle to interest him in preventive medicine.

It seems that the doctor sees the obvious need for biochemistry in his care of patients. This is clear at every turn, whether in medicine or surgery. Not so the preventive aspects. Faced by a patient who is already diseased, it is the exceptional man who looks toward prevention.*

The same holds true for the social and behavioral aspects of medicine. By and large the doctor is not interested in them.

This comparison between the success of the biochemistry department and the relative failure of that of preventive medicine suggests that the mere institution of a department of behavioral science in the medical school will not, of itself, remedy our problem. Likewise, it will not of itself suffice to put the medical school back into the University as Wedgwood implored us to do. The clinic must come to recognize the need.

A word about the relation of the growth of knowledge in behavioral science to the teaching of it. The newer understanding emerging from experimental neurophysiology, psychology, and sociology is prodigious. The whole curriculum could be crammed by interesting, pertinent observations. A difficulty of teaching the hard sciences has been the matter of selecting what should be taught. The behavioral sciences now face this same problem.

Professor Whittemore and Mr. Katan had a further comment on the addition of behavioral science as a subject in the curriculum.

Shall we operate on the assumption that this new addition in the curriculum is *not* and should not be just any new technical subject related with or added to the future medical practice, but a fundamental science encompassing all professions concerned with the alarming dehumanization of our exploded society? Would this not impregnate and change the whole curriculum?

We favor [this] alternative and believe that it is the role of this conference to rise above the daily contingency of personnel problems, transcend the many and enriching personal experiences, so as to draw general guidelines of a much needed blueprint. This is what we mean by getting beyond argument.

The several quotations from Wedgwood through Quarton

* The lack of interest in the preventive aspect of health care, which is so much a part of pediatrics, is believed by many to account for the relative shortage of pediatricians at the present time.

provide an abundance of ideas for what might be done to bring behavioral science into medicine. The participants, however, reached no consensus, no decisions, and there were no recommendations. Time did not permit.

The Endicott House Study also closed with many matters unsettled and limited recommendations, but the situations at the end of the two studies were not analogous. The Endicott House Study showed clearly that medical schools had made no preparation to receive the bright, better educated young students who are now graduating from many colleges. For these new students to be forced through the old medical curriculum with all its repetition is profligate of their time. They could easily encompass an enlightened medical curriculum in three years. The old courses in anatomy and biochemistry could be jettisoned. Many students are also well versed in physiology. A new more comprehensive course in pathology was recommended by Dr. Ivan Bennett to constitute the first year. Throughout the curriculum, experimentation and innovation were to be emphasized. The Endicott House Study did not have time, however, to consider several matters, including the education of women, sex education, the role of group practice in a medical school, the need for Negro physicians, ancillary personnel, administrators, and a new person in medicine—a systems engineer.

As this monograph is going to press, the Interdisciplinary Study of the Graduate Phase of Medical Education has been held. In the seven days of that Study, again there was not sufficient time to examine several of these problems. This third Study, however, closed triumphantly with a sweeping recommendation regarding the health needs of the nation—namely, adequate planning and support from the Federal Government, not to be counted in millions, but in billions of dollars. The problems of the graduate curriculum and the question of what to do with Medicare fees were as naught compared with the big problem of physician shortage and the urgent need for care of people in the Inner Cities, care for the people who at present receive no medical attention. These problems were considered by the Endicott House Study and the new medical schools recommended, but nothing, truly nothing, has been done. The sorry tale told by Dr. Child regarding the efforts to start a new school at the University of Michigan is an example. The delays that MIT and Harvard have had to face in forming an innovative medical school, because of faculty indecision, are another example. The need is urgent and it is the profession's obligation to get moving.

How do I view all of this? How can this all be pulled together? The several recommendations regarding teaching behavioral science in college, in a new department of behavioral science in the medical faculty, and Dr. Bond's approach to getting departments of medicine involved in behavioral science, are all to the good. Unfortunately, Dr. Bond's suggestion regarding the way to interest departments of medicine in behavioral science will take years to achieve what is needed. It should be put into action, nonetheless, because it will help; but by itself, it is not nearly enough. The teacher training and innovations advised by Dr. Quarton are also good, but how are they to be accomplished?

The only way to wrap up all these good ideas is by Dr. Quarton's third suggestion, the one originally proposed by the Endicott House Study—namely, new experimental schools of three years' duration. These could be set up forthwith and at minimal expense. Let's get on with it.

Participants

ANTHROPOLOGY

BOYD IRVEN DEVORE

Associate Professor of Anthropology, Harvard University, William James Hall, Cambridge, Massachusetts 02138

ARCHITECTURE

ROGER KATAN

Environmental Designer, Planning Consultant, 315 East 116th Street, New York, New York 10032

HISTORY

WILLIAM L. LANGER

Coolidge Professor of History, Emeritus, 1 Berkeley Street, Cambridge, Massachusetts 02138

INTERNAL MEDICINE

JOHN C. BECK

Professor of Medicine, McGill University, Royal Victoria Hospital, Montreal, 2, Canada

PHILIP K. BONDY

C.N.H. Long Professor, Department of Internal Medicine, Yale University School of Medicine, 333 Cedar Street, New Haven, Connecticut 06510

JAMES P. DIXON

President, Antioch College, Yellow Springs, Ohio 45387

ALEXANDER LEAF *

Jackson Professor of Clinical Medicine, Massachusetts General Hospital, Boston, Massachusetts 02114

AUSTIN S. WEISBERGER

Professor of Medicine, Western Reserve University, Cleveland, Ohio 44106

LAW

DAVID L. BAZELON

Chief Judge, United States Court of Appeals, Washington, DC 20001

LITERATURE

REED WHITTEMORE

National Institute of Public Affairs, 1001 Connecticut Avenue NW, Washington, DC 20036

NEUROLOGY

CHARLES D. ARING

Professor of Neurology, Cincinnati General Hospital, Cincinnati, Ohio 45229

PEDIATRICS

SALLY PROVENCE

Director, Child Development Unit, Child Study Center, Yale University, 333 Cedar Street, New Haven, Connecticut 06511

RALPH J. WEDGWOOD

Professor of Pediatrics, University of Washington, Seattle, Washington 98105

PHYSICS

JERROLD ZACHARIAS *

Institute Professor, Department of Physics, Massachusetts Institute of Technology, Cambridge, Massachusetts 02139

PSYCHIATRY

JOSE BARCHILON

Clinical Professor of Psychiatry, Colorado General Hospital, 4200 East Ninth Avenue, Denver, Colorado 80220

SAMUEL BARONDES

Assistant Professor of Psychiatry and Molecular Biology, Albert Einstein College of Medicine, Eastchester Road and Morris Park Avenue, Bronx, New York 10461

GRETE BIBRING *

Clinical Professor of Psychiatry, Emerita, Harvard Medical School, 47 Garden Street, Cambridge, Massachusetts 02138

DOUGLAS D. BOND *

Professor of Psychiatry, Western Reserve University, Cleveland, Ohio 44106

LEON EISENBERG

Professor of Child Psychiatry, The Johns Hopkins Hospital, Baltimore, Maryland 21205

DANIEL X. FREEDMAN

Professor of Psychiatry, The University of Chicago, 950 East 59th Street, Chicago, Illinois 60637

David Hamburg

Professor of Psychiatry, Stanford University School of Medicine, Palo Alto, California 94304

L. Douglas Lenkoski

Professor of Psychiatry, University Hospitals of Cleveland, Cleveland, Ohio 44106

Fritz C. Redlich

Professor of Psychiatry, Yale University School of Medicine, 333 Cedar Street, New Haven, Connecticut 06511

Vernon Rowland

Associate Professor of Psychiatry, University Hospitals of Cleveland, Cleveland, Ohio 44106

Gardner Quarton *

Psychiatrist, Chief of Stanley Cobb Laboratories, Massachusetts General Hospital, Boston, Massachusetts 02114

Benson R. Snyder *

Psychiatrist-in-Chief, Massachusetts Institute of Technology, Cambridge, Massachusetts 02139

Albert J. Solnit

Professor of Pediatrics and Psychiatry, Child Study Center, Yale University, 333 Cedar Street, New Haven, Connecticut 06511

Alan Stone

Director of Resident Education, McLean Hospital, Waltham, Massachusetts 02154

George Tarjan

Program Director, Department of Mental Retardation, The Neuropsychiatric Institute, UCLA Center for the Health Sciences, Los Angeles, California 90024

PSYCHOBIOLOGY

Seymour S. Kety

Chief, Laboratory of Clinical Science, National Institute of Mental Health, Bethesda, Maryland 20014

PSYCHOLOGY

Howard F. Hunt

Professor of Psychology, Department of Psychiatry, College of Physicians and Surgeons of Columbia University, New York, New York 10032

David Shakow

Chief, Laboratory of Psychology, National Institute of Mental Health, Bethesda, Maryland 20014

SOCIOLOGY

ROBERT STRAUS

Chairman, Department of Behavioral Science, University of Kentucky, Lexington, Kentucky 40506

SURGERY

ROBERT A. CHASE

Professor of Surgery, Stanford University School of Medicine, Palo Alto, California 94304

CHARLES G. CHILD, III *

Professor of Surgery, The University of Michigan, Ann Arbor, Michigan 48104

OLIVER COPE *

Professor of Surgery, Massachusetts General Hospital, Boston, Massachusetts 02114

One participant has withdrawn.

GUEST SPEAKERS

ANTHROPOLOGY

ARSENE BALIKCI

Professor of Anthropology, University of Montreal, Montreal, Canada

ANTHONY WALLACE

Professor of Anthropology, University of Pennsylvania, Philadelphia, Pennsylvania 19104

INTERNAL MEDICINE

COUNT GIBSON

Professor of Preventive Medicine, Tufts University School of Medicine, Medford, Massachusetts 02111

NEUROPHYSIOLOGY

HANS-LUKAS TEUBER

Professor of Psychology, Massachusetts Institute of Technology, Cambridge, Massachusetts 02139

PSYCHIATRY

ROBERT COLES

Research Psychiatrist to the Harvard University Health Services, 75 Mount Auburn Street, Cambridge, Massachusetts 02138

NORMAN PAUL

Assistant Clinical Professor of Psychiatry, Tufts University School of Medicine, Medford, Massachusetts 02111

MEDICAL STUDENTS

WILLIAM BENNETT
III Year Harvard Medical School, Boston, Massachusetts 02115

GORDON HARPER
III Year Harvard Medical School, Boston, Massachusetts 02115

JOSEPH YOUNGERMAN
III Year Harvard Medical School, Boston, Massachusetts 02115

OTHER GUESTS

ADMINISTRATION

JEROME B. WIESNER
Provost, Massachusetts Institute of Technology, Cambridge, Massachusetts 02139

EDITORIAL WRITER

ANN BARRETT
Houghton Mifflin Company, Boston, Massachusetts 02114

MEDICINE

HOWARD HIATT
Herrman Ludwig Blumgart Professor of Medicine, Beth Israel Hospital, Brookline, Massachusetts 02115

NEUROSURGERY

WILLIAM SWEET
Professor of Surgery, Massachusetts General Hospital, Boston, Massachusetts 02114

ORGANIZATIONS

ROBERT BERSON
Executive Director, Association of American Medical Colleges, 1501 New Hampshire Avenue, NW, Washington, DC 20036

ALAN PIFER
President, Carnegie Corporation of New York, 589 Fifth Avenue, New York, New York 10017

MARGARET MAHONEY
Associate Secretary and Executive Associate, Carnegie Corporation of New York, 589 Fifth Avenue, New York, New York 10017

FRITZ MOSHER
Executive Associate, Carnegie Corporation of New York, 589 Fifth Avenue, New York, New York 10017

PEDIATRICS

NATHAN TALBOT

Charles Wilder Professor of Pediatrics, Massachusetts General Hospital, Boston, Massachusetts 02114

SURGERY

OSCAR CREECH

Professor of Surgery, Tulane University School of Medicine, 1430 Tulane Avenue, New Orleans, Louisiana 70112

* STEERING COMMITTEE

GRETE BIBRING	ALEXANDER LEAF
DOUGLAS D. BOND, *Co-Chairman*	GARDNER QUARTON
CHARLES D. CHILD, III	BENSON R. SNYDER
OLIVER COPE, *Co-Chairman*	JERROLD ZACHARIAS, *Co-Chairman*

Dr. Ivan Bennett, Professor of Pathology, Dr. Joel Elkes, Professor of Psychiatry, both of Johns Hopkins University, and Dr. Eugene Stead, Professor of Medicine of Duke University, served as members of the Committee but were unable to attend the Study.

A Study of Behavioral Sciences in Medicine

COMMITTEE: DRS. BARONDES, BECK, BIBRING, COPE, KETY,
REDLICH, STRAUS AND WHITTEMORE

Report by Dr. Beck

THIS GROUP has viewed as its task the attempt to place the final "behavioral sciences brick" into what is at present an acceptable curriculum in most medical schools. Placing this brick would permit the opening of many curricula to bolder experimentation in their design. Although some members of the group felt that this Report is reactionary, the majority, I believe, considered it moderately conservative. We have attempted to define the interrelationships among the natural, behavioral, and clinically applied sciences, and the latter category, we would emphasize, includes both psychiatry and the major clinical subject areas.

I. Objectives

To increase the awareness of the student, faculty and the medical community to the psychological and social aspects of health and disease, and to enrich the empathy between physician and patient. By so doing, contributions to the advancement of knowledge in these areas will accrue, emphasizing their importance and helping to motivate and guide appropriate community activity.

These objectives can be reached through meaningful involvement with selected concepts and data from the several behavioral sciences, which will provide an understanding of:

1. The interdependence of biological, psychological, social and environmental phenomena in determining
   a. the pathogenesis, distribution, diagnosis and management of specific disease processes,

b. the potentialities for prevention or modification of disease, and

c. the beliefs, attitudes and values associated with human response to illness in general and to specific forms of disease.

2. *A historical perspective* and a perspective of comparative cultures as bases for considering the impact of technological and social change on

a. the nature of contemporary and future society, and

b. the nature of contemporary and future medical science and forms of medical care.

3. *Processes of communication* and human relationships that are basic to the interaction of health personnel with patients and with each other, and the application of communication skills to activities in the medical setting.

4. *The social structure* of universities, hospitals and other health organizations and the factors governing the organization and distribution of health resources to the community.

In delineating the objectives, we must emphasize that contributions to the advancement of knowledge in the behavioral sciences is imperative for the success of their introduction into the Undergraduate curriculum. These contributions would help to motivate and guide appropriate community activities in gaining additional understanding of many of the problems that now confront us clinically.

In the following section, we attempted to define in broad terms the body of knowledge that we think encompasses the behavioral sciences; this task obviously implied that the group felt that such a body of knowledge at present exists.

II. A Body of Knowledge

The body of knowledge that can be encompassed by the term *Behavioral Sciences* can be subdivided, for a variety of purposes, into: *A*. Neural-behavioral sciences, *B*. Individual psychology, and *C*. Social-cultural sciences. These divisions are not rigid; they overlap, and interdependence exists between them. Their content may be defined as follows:

A. NEURAL-BEHAVIORAL SCIENCES

Physiologic psychology Behavioral genetics
Chemical psychology Embryologic and morphologic
Behavioral pharmacology development of the nervous system

B. INDIVIDUAL PSYCHOLOGY

A study of personality and personality development, including the concepts of affect, memory, learning, motivational drives, communication, consciousness and language.

These would be presented as a series of observations, and in the theoretic formulation of these concepts, use would be made of the prevailing schools of thought concerning their integration. Of these the most prevalent is psychoanalytic theory, although others provide interesting although as yet incomplete formulation (e.g., S-R theory, learning theory, etc.).

C. SOCIAL-CULTURAL SCIENCES

Anthropology	History (organization of man)
Sociology	Economics
Ethology	Political Science
	Demography

These should include the development of concepts of dynamic social change; historical and cultural relativity; social class and social stratification, including analysis of social systems; role; functioning of small and large groups and organizations.

The Committee concerned itself at some length with consideration of methods whereby the importance of the behavioral sciences might be conveyed to university students in general and to medical students in particular. It was concluded that there must be a mechanism developed at the college, or perhaps even at the precollege level, for the interdisciplinary-interdepartmental preprofessional training of students around the general subject area of Man, His Environment and Society. This should not be just another interdisciplinary course, but should have as an important integral total involvement of the student by actual *doing*. Repeated emphasis must be placed on the abolition of single-discipline courses for this purpose, with the aim of developing a program crossing the traditional subject lines, which would produce relevantly educated graduates, ready, if they happen to become medical students, to deal humanely and intelligently with their patients. In projecting an extension of this into the medical school environment, it was felt that the best teaching model would be Columbia Point or its equivalent.

This view was dictated because we felt that a medical motivation must be introduced during the medical school experience in order that maximum return might be obtained from the student's point of view. In contrast to the subject title above, one might propose for this section, as title, The Medical Student—rather than Man—His Environment and Society. In considering course content, method, and techniques of presentation at the medical school, it was felt that the choice among many methods of teaching depended in part on the individual teacher, the student, and the particular university or medical school milieu. Three conditions must be met:

1. Involvement. The student should be involved with a major subdivision within medicine, such as Internal Medicine or Surgery.

2. The involvement must provide *identification* with physicians, using physicians in a narrower sense, and not solely with psychiatrists.

3. Techniques must be relatively simple at the early stage, since there is inherent danger in placing the student in a complex situation with which he is not equipped to deal.

For situations in which the student could gain perspective on his or her eventual role, four suggestions are presented:

1. There should be developed in the first and perhaps subsequent years within the medical school a mechanism by which the student can go to someone within Faculty who has a broad understanding of medical education in general and particularly of the psychosocial factors in this educational experience.

2. Extensive discussion revolved around the unstructured, or T-type or sensitivity group, and it was felt that it might be a useful experimental model for some medical schools to use in an attempt to gain a greater understanding of the student, the student's interplay with his confreres and with his teachers, in the hope that the student might gain greater understanding of himself. This might well make the suggestion in Section I (A Tutorial System) more effective.

3. Small group interplay could be developed about specific subject areas with which the medical student comes in contact early in his medical career. A good example of this would be the intractably ill or the dying patient.

4. The development of small group interplay around a case. In order to make such an experience meaningful, it would necessitate certain recapitulation of basic, essential information, and in addition would involve the development of skill in Interviewing Techniques early in the medical school experience, since the success or failure of any of these suggestions is in large part dependent on this skill.

III. Content, Method, Relevance

In considering content, method and relevance in the present educational systems, we would recommend the development of an interdepartmental, interdisciplinary course in the pre-professional training of physicians as well as the other professions. This teaching program should be centered about the heading, Man, Environment and Society.

IV. Strategy

A. For the Introduction of Behavioral Science into the Medical School

It is ultimately desired that each medical school will contain an autonomous Department of Behavioral Science. It is recognized that introduction and development of such a department may not be immediately possible, but rather that individual medical schools have different needs and potentialities for its development. This section will describe: *1.* The nature of the ultimate and ideal behavioral science department, and *2.* Some alternative strategies for the gradual development of such departments in the different medical schools.

THE NATURE OF A DEPARTMENT OR DIVISION OF BEHAVIORAL SCIENCE

Goal. The Department of Behavioral Science should have as its goal both the teaching of behavioral science relevant to medical practice and research and also the teaching of the students in clinical settings of a behavioral approach to all medical patients.

The need for a separate department. A separate department or division is desirable for reasons of prestige. A chair supported by the university should be present in each medical school, and departmental funds should also be available as in other more conventional departments. The existence of a discrete department will also provide for the opportunity to have a substantial number of people interested in the same type of approach housed together, so that they may stimulate each other and, because of the self-generating nature of such interactions, evolve new teaching methods and research objectives, which might not occur to individuals in such disciplines who are housed in a nonmedical setting. The Committee recognized the flux occurring with respect to departmental structures in many medical schools, and recognizes the inherent disadvantages of departmental barriers. We were endeavoring to create an environment that would permit identification of the behavioral scientist with his own area, recognizing that every effort should be made to prevent the isolation of such a department from the medical school proper, or from the behavioral science area within the university as a whole.

Specific recommendations about faculty members. Such a department should include:

1. People trained in special behavioral sciences, particularly sociology, anthropology and experimental psychology.
2. Psychiatrists specially trained in psychotherapy or another behavioral science.
3. Internists and surgeons who have had special training either in psychotherapy or in one of the other behavioral areas.

It is believed that the people with medical or psychiatric backgrounds are of great importance in transmitting the information developed in behavioral sciences to the medical students, both in formal lectures and also in more clinical and individual settings. It is felt that the existence of a department with which these faculty members feel closely allied will provide them with the needed support so that they can emphasize as their speciality the behavioral approach rather than more conventional specialized approaches (hematology, gastroenterology, etc.).

B. For the Evolution of a Department or Division of Behavioral Sciences in a Medical School

In most medical schools, departments of behavioral sciences cannot spring up overnight: there must be a process of gradual evolution. Such evolution would have as its two major characteristics:

1. The development of personnel who were acquainted both with behavioral sciences and medicine.
2. The development of attitudes within the medical and hospital communities that would allow such people the dignity and importance that their roles command.

Some medical schools, like those of the University of Kentucky and the University of Florida, have attempted to establish independent departments of behavioral sciences; other schools of medicine, like Stanford's, have developed to a conspicuous extent Departments of Psychiatry that have incorporated within them behavioral scientists; and most medical schools have undertaken to encourage liaison between departments of psychiatry and departments of medicine and surgery. There are, therefore, evidences for beginnings in the direction felt to be desirable.

The important steps in the development of personnel and attitudes in the medical community are as follows:

1. Sending out from established departments of medicine and surgery respected young people who will be encouraged to train extensively either in a behavioral science like sociology or in clinical psychiatry. These people would then return to their home department and, because of their familiarity, be in a position to introduce what they have learned to their colleagues: much as other specialists are currently generated (e.g., sending internists to a department of biochemistry as preparation for studying the biochemistry of some metabolic disorder).

2. Psychiatrists should be encouraged to temporarily leave their department for study in university departments of behavioral science, like sociology, and then return to their departments to stimulate their colleagues in a broader picture of the behavioral approach.

3. Departments of psychiatry and also departments of medicine and surgery should be encouraged to welcome highly selected behavioral scientists for a period of several years of study within their departments. These people would be primarily trained in their own behavioral discipline, and would then be encouraged to learn more about the practical problems of human care traditionally assigned to the physician. These people could then use their own techniques to generate research and new ideas about patient care, and could ultimately supplement the physician-behavioral scientist in evolving a core of people committed to this approach.

Evolution of Students' Attitudes during Medical School

COMMITTEE: JUDGE BAZELON, DRS. BOND, BONDY, DEVORE, EISENBERG, HUNT, ROWLAND, SNYDER AND TARJAN

Report by Dr. Bondy

THESE REMARKS represent an attempt to explore changes that occur in the attitudes of students toward patients and social processes during the course of their medical school career. It is based on certain assumptions and observations. The assumptions are:

1. That students decide to enter the medical profession because of their involvement, in varying degrees, with human suffering. In the present climate of scientific financial support, the student whose major interest is in pure biological sciences is likely to find it both easier and financially more advantageous to seek a degree in one of the basic sciences than to attempt to obtain an MD degree. The social and economic advantages that once attracted people to a career in medicine seem much less lustrous today. Therefore, in most instances an important factor leading a student to enter a medical school must be his interest in human disease and in the opportunity for helping sick patients or preventing the development of sickness. In support of this contention, Solkoff and Markowitz (J Med Educ 42:195-199, March, 1967) find that psychological tests show a higher score for "humanitarianism" in medical students than in law students.

2. That students entering medical school have already been exposed in considerable depth to the basic material of the social and behavioral sciences. This exposure includes formal high school or college course work, reading in novels and biography,

and personal experiences, which may include travel and work in slum or depressed areas.

Changes in Attitudes

At some time during their medical school or postdoctoral training program, many medical students or young physicians assume attitudes that reflect failure to apply this knowledge to clinical situations or even a desire to "divorce themselves" from these attitudes. This tendency has been documented by Eron (Eron, L.D.: J Med Educ 30:559, 1955), who found that medical students tended to become more cynical and less idealistic as they passed from their first to their fourth year of study. In contrast to this, although not necessarily in contradiction to it, is Snyder's finding (J Med Educ 42:213, March, 1967) that medical students tended to become more oriented to the demands of society during their medical school career. Apparently the way in which medical students' attitudes changed depended in part on their experiences in medical school and in part on the attitudes they had developed and the experiences they had had prior to entering medical school. It seems likely, therefore, that their lack of appreciation for social and behavioral components in medical practice does not reflect failure of exposure but rather some influence or set of influences in the medical school that leads some students to minimize the importance of these aspects of their prior training.

FACTORS THAT LEAD TO CHANGES

A number of the factors that lead to these changes can be suggested:

1. The need of the student to develop a protective carapace so that he can tolerate the unpleasant experiences of the clinic. At some time in his professional training, each student must learn to handle the emotional disturbance caused by his patients' suffering without allowing it to overwhelm him. He will often be confronted with tragedy he cannot alleviate or with pain that he must tolerate or even himself inflict. If he allows himself to be too upset by these necessary aspects of the healing art, he will not be able to function effectively. One of his earliest tasks in the clinic will be to apply dispassionate, intellectual processes to studying disturbing, painful or even disgusting

aspects of human suffering. Unless he can learn this dispassionate attitude, he will never be an effective physician. On the other hand, somewhere along the line he must develop a balanced attitude that does not exclude a recognition of the social, behavioral and psychiatric factors that make the patient a person rather than simply an intellectual problem in disordered physiology. The development of this balance takes time and experience. The first step usually represents an overshoot in the direction of "toughness" and cynicism.

2. In developing his attitudes towards patients, the student will pattern himself to considerable extent on the faculty and more senior doctors in training. If these preceptors have not themselves as yet developed a mature attitude and are indifferent or skeptical about the importance of social and behavioral factors, the student will tend to reinforce his tough attitude. This is particularly likely to be so if the older physicians with whom he is in contact in his training suggest that it will be unpalatable to them if the student considers psychiatric, social or behavioral influences when he discusses his patient.

3. If the faculty is unaware of the adjustments that the student must undergo, they are likely to be insensitive to the students' needs and attitudes. The faculty themselves may continue to present a facade of self-assurance that rejects the importance of factors outside the technical or organic aspects of medicine. Commonly this attitude expresses itself in a humorous denigration of the psychosocial and behavioral aspects of medicine. Laughter is a powerful weapon, which can overwhelm all but the most secure student.

4. The increasing (and desirable) expansion of full-time teachers in the clinical faculty tends to develop a somewhat different approach in university medicine from that of most private physicians. As a result, the student sees medicine from a particular economic and social orientation, which may not reflect the realities of private medical practice. It is difficult to develop and demonstrate the ideal relationship between the physician, the patient and his family under these circumstances.

To Encourage Desirable Attitudes

If these considerations are appropriate, it should be possible to encourage and protect the desirable attitudes:

1. By recognizing, as part of the medical school admission policy, that exposure in depth to college courses in the behavioral sciences is desirable along with exposure to the "hard" sciences. It might be appropriate to recommend some course work in sociology, anthropology, or normal psychology as part of the premedical curriculum.

2. By organizing the curriculum in such a way that students may take courses in the behavioral sciences in the university, and by encouraging them to do so.

3. By exposing students early in the first year of medical school to contact with patients and emphasizing, during this contact, the behavioral or social aspects of the patients' problems, as well as the physical and medical considerations.

4. By encouraging the participation of faculty members in study and research in behavioral aspects of medicine. This includes recognizing such study as appropriate for scientists who are contributing members of the medical faculty, and rewarding activity in this area by promotion and administrative assignments on the same basis as faculty members concerned more particularly with physicochemical aspects of disease.

5. By introducing into the clinical curriculum a constant awareness of the importance of these factors. This awareness can be promoted only by constant encouragement by the senior faculty—by discussion, questioning and sympathetic promotion of the exploration of these facets of patient care.

6. By helping the students to understand their own reactions toward patients. Some of this understanding can be conveyed during introductory courses in psychiatry.

7. By providing an opportunity to learn about the methods of delivering medical care, in which context the relations between the physician and his patient may be explored fruitfully. Such a course would also logically consider economic, social and political influences affecting the relationship between doctor and patients, and the circumstances under which patients seek and accept medical care.

8. By exploiting, within the medical center, many factors of interest to behavioral scientists that affect the interrelations of students, faculty, patients, and the administrative structure of the school and the hospital. These interactions could be exploited constructively by using the medical school itself as a model to be observed by the students, under guidance from social scientists. Many schools use questionnaires and interviews with students to guide them in making administrative or curricular decisions. More direct participation in some of these decision-making processes, with analysis of some of the factors involved, might help orient the students more constructively toward the realities of medical economics and care in our society.

The major justification for a medical school is its ability to educate physicians capable of rendering and promoting the best possible medical care to patients. In addition to the technical problems with which the student must become familiar, he must also come to understand the economic, social, psychiatric and other behavioral influences that affect his ability to function as a physician. Education in these areas does not require any major modification of the medical school curriculum, but it does require full exploitation of the positive experiences and opportunities afforded by the milieu of a medical center.

Study of Human Behavior

COMMITTEE: DRS. ARING, BOND, CHASE, HAMBURG, LANGER,
LEAF, PROVENCE, SOLNIT, AND STONE

Report by Drs. Solnit and Provence

*Illustrations by Drs. Aring, Hamburg, Leaf,
Provence, and Solnit*

THE CHANGING CONDITIONS and content of medical care and the desperate need to modify the educational opportunities for medical students are emphatically joined in the study of human behavior. The behavioral sciences in medical education have posed a complex set of difficulties and a crucial opportunity. In the following proposal, the service-centered study and understanding of human behavior and development in a large variety of settings are viewed as an aim that can be achieved most fruitfully by the student through his helping and caring for other people in a manner that matches the student's interests and capacities to the needs and interests of the persons being helped.

A. The Medical Student

There is a great need to build into the medical student's education opportunities and experiences that keep alive his scientific curiosity and interest in people. How can we keep the student a member of society while he is in training? How can we correct the errors of the present system of medical education, in which the important human characteristics of the student and the patient are largely overlooked? How and when can we involve him with people in an effective and not contrived way?

Some of the principles and assumptions that underlie the attempt to answer the questions above are:

110

1. The student should be encouraged to assume an active role in influencing and determining his own training.

2. He needs to be active in his area of concern and future responsibility, namely in the care of people.

3. An appropriate experience with people should be made available to him at the very beginning of his medical education.

4. The extent of his involvement and responsibility will depend on his level of competence, which should be judged by medical faculty members who know of his previous education and current readiness to assume such responsibility.

5. The involvement with people in the first year will be required of all students except, as Professor Zacharias said, those who do not want it. This attitude differs from designating it as an *elective* or *required* experience.

6. Considerable diversity and individual variation is to be expected among the students, which imposes a greater demand for flexibility in the curriculum and for knowledge of the student by the faculty.

7. In regard to the method of education, there was general agreement that both *a.* the "mealworm" concept, in which the student is helped to find a bit of nature and learn to ask and answer his own questions about it, and *b.* the communication of information and attitudes from faculty to student via lectures, seminars, demonstrations, audio-visual aids etc. are needed. Most present curricula suffer from overdoing type *b.* It is important to provide both types of educational experience in a proportion that will support the student's learning.

8. The study of human behavior includes the assumption of expecting a continuing development and change in the field, not merely the application of what is now known. This applies to all other areas of medicine as well. Since knowledge will increase and needs and methods will change, it is crucial that we stimulate *attitudes* and approaches that help prepare the student for his future life as a physician.

9. It is deemed *absolutely essential* that there be a system through which a close relationship between a student and one or more faculty can be developed: it will not be possible to individualize the learning experience in a safe and meaningful way without close contact between student and faculty members.

B. The Program

The active engagement of students in the study of man, his environment and his behavior should be planned according to the interests of the student and the opportunities presented by his community and faculty. This suggested course of action-study is an attempt to respond to the manifest interest and self-initiated activities of college students in the social and health problems of our society, and to the conviction that medical education requires curriculum revamping and innovation in studying human behavior and development. In this proposal, it is assumed that this course of action-study should ideally take place in the first four years of college, enabling medical schools to introduce their students to clinical medicine, the assessment and care of patients, in a sensible fashion in the first year of medical studies. However, it is also assumed that if the student has not had an adequate course of action-study in human behavior in the undergraduate years, he should have it available in his first year of medical school. It is further assumed that the introduction to clinical medicine would incorporate advanced exercises in the study of human behavior as it relates to medical care and research. As a vehicle for implementing this proposal, it is suggested that a Council on the Study of Human Behavior be organized and that this Council be made up of student and faculty representatives.

COUNCIL ON THE STUDY OF HUMAN BEHAVIOR

Social Aspects   *Biological Aspects*

Field Experiences
Laboratory Experiences
Seminars
Supervision
(e.g., Phillips Brooks House, Dwight Hall)

Field

Schools	Other social agencies	Primate labs
Hospitals	Prisons	Animal labs
Settlement houses	Court clinics	Foreign land projects
Nursery schools	Foster homes	(Anthropology field
Day care program	Teenage groups	study)
Half-way house	Migratory labor corps	Neurophysiology

Seminars

Seminar: *a*) Introductory   Faculty: Clinical
         b) Advanced   Nonclinical
Student forum, with budget   Faculty advisor

In order for this program, of a Council on the Study of Human Behavior, to work effectively, it would require enthusiasm and commitment, as well as distributed responsibility for its execution, by three groups. The students' interest and influence on the program is essential. The faculty's interest, energy and competence should be assured. Those responsible for the hospital and community settings into which students would enter in an active responsible manner should have the option of participating and hopefully would only agree to collaborate if it makes sense to them and represents some aspects of their own hopes for the future of medical education and the advancement of the behavioral sciences.

We assume that students will require assistance in representing the University's effort to reach out, find and enable certain persons or families to help themselves. These persons or families are those who are either unable to plan and organize themselves to benefit from being members of our society or who have characteristically isolated themselves from contact with the resources in their community. The students are to elect the environment and the people with whom they wish to engage, selecting from a range of situations that have been determined to offer realistic opportunities for such service in the particular community in which the university lives. These are service-learning situations for the students, which can be enriched by the interest, supervision, and intellectual content provided by the faculty of the university.

As already indicated, the Council on the Study of Human Behavior would be composed of student and faculty representatives. The student group would be drawn from undergraduate and graduate levels, including medical students. The faculty representatives would be drawn from the university at large, but should include qualified members of the clinical faculties, including experienced social workers.

The aim of such a course is to enable students to study man through helping him. The interests and capacities of the student and the needs of the person being helped should be matched in a rational and practical manner. The student's active interest and engagement should be an avenue to the inquiry into human behavior and development that enables the student to exploit seminar discussions and study of various aspects of man and his environment, with faculty taking its lead from the students in regard to the content and sequences of concepts and techniques being considered. Thus, we are not aiming at a comprehensive or systematic study of human behavior and development; rather we are aiming to help each student acquire self-awareness in his continuing study of man, an awareness of a range of conceptual frames of reference and techniques useful for understanding and studying human behavior, and an experience in how to proceed in the scholarly study of man in the context of the traditional humanitarian medical alliance of one man helping another.

In the seminar, student forums, reading and experimental exploration of the bodies of knowledge that are relevant to this action-study, it is assumed that the students will have access to faculty members in the behavioral sciences as well as in the humanities and clinical sciences. Thus concepts and methods derived from anthropology, ethology, history, law, psychiatry, psychoanalysis, social psychology, and sociology and other disciplines can be used to illuminate and analyze the student's field experiences and to promote his ability to conceptualize and actively acquire critical knowledge about man, his behavior, and his environment.

The time requirements for such a course would be a minimum of half-day a week for a year, including field and seminar work and supervision.

Among the advantages of this proposal is that of recruiting into medicine certain students for whom the study of human behavior is compelling, and that of recruiting and preparing more faculty members who can help to establish, develop and man the new medical schools that are essential for the present and future health needs of this nation.

ILLUSTRATION: *Dr. Aring*

A delegate (or delegation) of Student and Faculty Council in charge of studies in Human Behavior would interview every student to determine his interests and his stage of development in relation to the program. He would be assigned a supervisor to whom he could report when a problem arose.

I will select as an example of a community agency (in Cincinnati), the School for Crippled Children, a facility in the Elementary School System, located a few blocks from the Medical Center. Here are taught youngsters too crippled to enter the regular schools. They are bussed to and from school. I would guess the total population of crippled children to be somewhere around 50 to 75. The reasons for crippling are myriad and include, among others, birth injury, syringomyelia, muscular dystrophy and other familial neuromuscular disorders.

The student electing the School for Crippled Children as his endeavor could devote some attention to the specific problems, current and projected, that involved a child and his family by reason of his crippling. The attitudes developed by the child, the family and society through restriction of movement and differences highlighted by an inability to partake in sports and other healthy projects, and the compensatory derivatives and defenses would concern him, not alone by way of his little student but in general. During his term of service, which would preferably occupy the year, he might serve as a tutor (or assistant teacher) to his pupil, one of several supporting roles that might be considered. An enduring relationship might sometimes result.

It is expected that a medical student would become interested in learning in some depth about the disease or disorder that had caused the crippling; one could even imagine the development of a research interest about it.

ILLUSTRATION: *Dr. Hamburg*

An illustrative approach toward a first-year medical school course in the study of human behavior.

Procedure: Survey a variety of university departments regarding their interest in participation.

    a. Appropriate settings for student involvement—i.e., is there a functional role for the student in some setting familiar to a given department? Such settings might include wards, clinics, schools, social agencies.

    b. Faculty participation—is there anyone who would be interested in working with the students in this course in order to ensure that the activity would have educational substance?

Diversity of faculty participation, e.g.:

1. On-site supervision and collaboration
2. Seminar
3. Guided readings

Example of one setting for such activity:

A day-care center for emotionally disturbed children. The student comes to the center one afternoon per week for at least one quarter, preferably longer. He is assigned one child upon whom to concentrate his attention. His task is to form a dependable relationship with this child in whatever ways seem appropriate to him, with the guidance of an on-site supervisor, the clinical director of the day-care center. He will also interview the parents of the child along lines worked out in advance with his supervisor.

When his relationship with the child has advanced to a suitable point, he may take the child on special outings. Supervisory discussions precede and follow such outings. The student makes a record of the child's behavior on each occasion.

Every second week, the student meets with his faculty mentor (probably not the same person as his on-site supervisor, though this would vary from one setting to another). Major issues of child development are discussed, arising largely out of the student's observations and questions. Readings on these issues are suggested and discussed. Such reading might include, for example, the following: relevant portions of the introductory child development textbooks by Stone and Church or by Mussen, Conger and Kagan; portions of Erickson's *Childhood and Society;* portions of Brown's *Social Psychology;* several of the research reviews in the Hoffman and Hoffman volume on recent research in child development; clinical papers by Bowlby, Solnit, Eisenberg, Kanner; primate development papers by DeVore, Jay, Hamburg, and Harlow.

There would be a monthly evening seminar in which several students engaged in similar projects would meet with their faculty mentor(s). On each occasion, one student would present his work. He would also provide a context based on his analysis of the relevant literature, a systematic comparison with at least one other similar project (e.g., another approach to treatment of the same kind of children), and suggestions for future inquiry.

ILLUSTRATIONS: *Dr. Leaf*

Specific Instances of Field Experience in Behavioral Study

Medical students could be assigned to various ambulatory or in-patient facilities in a general hospital during their first year. The pertinence to behavioral study of the experience in a social-action directed activity, which they elect, would be monitored by the Student-Faculty Council on Behavioral Study. Where the hospital facility does not provide from its own staff or faculty individuals qualified to supervise the student's experience, then the Council will designate an appropriate mentor.

1. IN AMBULATORY CLINIC

A. Ambulatory care in a hospital. Purpose of Study:
To allow a beginning medical student to examine how a hospital's outpatient service operates and to make suggestions for improvement of diagnostic and therapeutic services.

Procedure of Study: Student will collect data regarding how much time physicians spend with new and follow-up patients. Are patients satisfied with their contacts with physicians? How long does the initial diagnostic work-up take? Where are the bottlenecks? Does the student feel that good medical care and patient satisfaction are achieved in this facility? How could this be improved?

B. Case assignment. Purpose of Study:

To learn, by following an individual case, how well the care needs of the patient are met by the Ambulatory Clinic and what the role of family, or other social agencies is in supplementing and assisting the function of the Clinic.

Procedure of Study: Assign diabetic patient who is difficult to control to a student. Let student familiarize himself with the principles of diabetic management, dietary, pharmacological, etc. Let him see how adequately patient follows the prescription of Clinic doctor. What community facilities, visiting nurse, diet clinics, diabetic association facilities can contribute to the care of this patient? What has the disease done to the effectiveness of the patient as a citizen, at school, at work, etc? What suggestions can student offer to improve the Ambulatory Clinic care of diabetic patients?

2. MEDICAL INPATIENT

A. Case assignment, e.g., rheumatoid arthritis. Purpose of Study:

For student to direct patient to agencies in the community that will assist rehabilitation and care of patient during and after hospitalization.

Procedure of Study: Student will acquaint himself with the patient, her disease, her home environment. He will find out about follow-up visit facilities. He will learn what community agencies exist and how they may help his patient after leaving the hospital, social service, visiting nurses, domestic help, occupational therapy and rehabilitation service, welfare agencies and support. He will assist his patient to obtain the needed services. He will suggest other facilities that would help, and improvements in services of existing facilities.

ILLUSTRATION: *Dr. Provence*

Illustration of Student Activity—Yale Child Study Center

The Yale Child Study Center's Child Development Unit sees many infants and young children with a wide variety of problems of development, ranging from mild and transitory disturbances to severe impairments from biological and/or psychosocial causes. The presence of a nursery school of normal children provides an easily available setting in which the contrasts between the normal and abnormal child can be highlighted. The staff of child development and family specialists from pediatrics, psychology, social work, psychiatry, psychoanalysis, and education provides appropriate supervisors and resource people for the student, who can be related to the specific experience arranged for the student.

Of many possible examples, one frequently encountered is chosen as an example.

Patient: Johnny D. is a four-year-old boy with delayed speech, living in a third foster home and one in which there is no father. The question asked by the responsible agency—what is the cause of the delayed speech; is the child mentally retarded? brain damaged? etc.?

Objectives for the student:

1. To become aware of the complexity of speech development and the multiple factors that may influence it.

2. To provide (if appropriate) male companionship for a fatherless four-year-old boy and to evaluate this experience for himself and the child.

Procedure	*Topics (followed in depth according to student's interest)*
1. Observe and discuss the developmental assessment of the child, including differential diagnosis.	a. Methods of assessment (tests, etc.) b. Techniques of observing behavior and of recording observations
2. Visit the foster home with the social worker from the Division of Child Welfare. Make observations, preplanned, with supervision.	a. Selection of foster homes b. Function of Child Welfare Agencies c. Problems of child placement
3. Accompany Johnny and his foster mother to appointments in the medical center, necessary to the differential diagnosis, e.g., Hearing and Speech Center for audiometric examination, and the pediatric clinic.	a. Hearing, normal/abnormal, neurologic considerations, techniques of assessment b. The problem of anxiety in child and mother in regard to medical procedures c. The pediatric examination
4. Visit the child, at an interval to be selected, to be a companion.	a. Theory of interpersonal relationships b. Age appropriate activities of the child related to development c. Needs of fatherless child, etc.

ILLUSTRATION: *Dr. Solnit*

Study of Man, His Behavior, and His Environment

For those students at Yale University who are interested in working with disturbed children and their families, we would appoint a member of the child psychiatry faculty as supervisor. The supervisor would interview the students referred to him by the Council in order to determine the suitability of the Child Study Center's resources and the student's interests and capacities. In any one year, we would probably be able to take on four to six students whom we would ask to provide companionship and tutoring assistance for children aged eight to fourteen, with school learning difficulties and problems of impulse control. The children would probably be in psychiatric treatment, and the student would become a member of the child psychiatry team involved in caring for the child and his family. The student would be introduced as a college or medical student who could help the child learn how to overcome his problems by seeing him twice a week in his neighborhood, where he also would get to know the child's family, friends, neighbors and teachers. The child psychiatric aide would help the child by becoming friends with him and his family, playing with the child, helping him with his lessons, and taking him on planned trips to interesting and worthwhile places and events in the community. The child psychiatric aide would be supervised at least once every two weeks, or every week. He would be invited, his time permitting, to participate in child psychiatry conferences and to become familiar with the Child Study Center's activities and staff.

Since the school child's schedule is clear, the aide would plan to see him in the afternoon or evening. In addition to his regular supervisor, he would have easy access to social workers, pediatricians, psychologists and educators attached to the Center. As the student's experience and knowledge developed, and if he were interested in working in greater depth, there are children with problems of development, education and socializing that the student would work with in a variety of ways. This range of opportunities for the advanced student include research and therapy opportunities at the Child Study Center, in special settings in the community, and in the clinics and wards of the Department of Pediatrics.

Our Primary Purpose

COMMITTEE: DRS. BARCHILON, CHILD, FREEDMAN, KATAN,
LENKOSKI, QUARTON AND WEDGWOOD

Report by Drs. Child and Wedgwood

THE PRIMARY PURPOSE of a medical school in the past was to impart a closed body of knowledge or identifiable content requisite for a physician's function. This is no longer true. The primary purpose of medical education and training today is to develop differing problem-solving capabilities of diverse students in a particular environment with particular varieties of populations. It must be assumed that the relevant content in great part will be learned by the process of incidental as well as planned contact.

The best technique for the development of problem-solving capabilities is a modification of the case study method, which provides insight into not only the content and questions raised by the subject of study, but also into the nature and habits of thinking of the student.

The attitudes of a physician are an important function for medical education. These attributes are best developed through the case study method and are not solely the responsibility of any one discipline.

Many contributions of the physical, biological and behavioral sciences and humanities are relevant to medicine, and are properly university disciplines. These should be freely available to all students within a medical school, as well as to all students of any discipline within a university.

The behavioral sciences have a triple role in medical education. The knowledge of behavioral science acquired by the physician-teacher plays a role in planning the use of the case method to help students think clearly, evaluate evidence, and ask questions of nature. The knowledge of behavioral science acquired by both is effective in teaching psychiatry and social medicine. The ability to evaluate evidence and ask questions of nature is equally important here. Behavioral science deserves a role in medical schools of the associated university exactly like that of biochemistry, which makes available lectures, seminars, laboratory experience in depth, and teachers as models. This use of behavioral science is not in conflict with other uses, but is complementary.

There are also contributions of clinical science and faculties that constitute resources for a university. These should also be made available to all university students.

The end product of such a learning process is an individual who can continue to recognize the human qualities of man and derive through such understanding the pertinent questions that need to be resolved.

We have been discussing how to put behavioral science (and the humanities) into medical education. This is inappropriate; we should be discussing how to put a medical school into a university, which contains in aggregate these disciplines. The implementation of these goals requires medical schools to change from a closed educational system, to a new role—that of an educational resource in a university. Solution requires consideration of those details and relationships demanded by the concept of a truly "Open University," one of whose facets constitutes the resources of a medical school—and its health services.

The major contribution, the focal point of the medical school in this new role, might be to provide a single unit course, which would be the sole prerequisite for all subsequent medical course work. This unit would emphasize in a carefully structured manner, with trained and committed faculty, problem-solving techniques through the case study method on patients. The prerequisites for the course would be varied, but should require some experience in depth in the scientific method. The unit and its elaborations would be available not only for future physicians, but also possibly for many students of other disciplines.

If one can consider the process of medical education today as a continuum extending from at least high school through at least residency and board certification, then with appropriate faculty guidance, using the graduate school system and utilizing flexible breadth and depth requirements, the remainder of the education-training process could be freely elective—limited only by licensure and certification requirements, and these too can be changed.

Comments on Study of Behavioral Science in Medicine

DR. SHAKOW

The Task of the Conference

OBVIOUSLY THE major goal of the Conference was seen differently by various members of the group. At one time or another it appeared to me that these four goals were expressed:

1. Socialization and humanization of the physician,
2. The behavioral sciences as basic disciplines necessary for the full teaching of medicine,
3. The medical school as a part of the broader university setting and of the behavioral sciences in the combined set-up, and
4. The narrower proposition of Judge Bazelon relating to making the medically trained psychiatrist adequate to deal with important social issues.

Let me elaborate somewhat on each of these.

The argument for the socialization and humanization of the physician in training arises from recent developments. Advances in medicine have tended to direct the students' energies to areas that derive their prestige largely from laboratory work. The recent advances in neurophysiology, molecular biology, and other basic sciences have had the effect of emphasizing process rather than the person. This has resulted in the impersonalization of the physician as physician. Many medical men who come in direct clinical contact with patients believe that it is necessary to inject into medicine a more social, a more personal and generally a more human approach. This attitude is also reflected in Walter Goodman's recent article in the *NY Times Magazine* Section (Oct. 12, 1966) and the earlier books of Carter, Greenberg, Lasagna, and Gross.

123

Those who held that the Conference was directed toward the consideration of the behavioral sciences and their place in the basic medical curriculum presented a somewhat different argument. They indicated that, in earlier years, there had been a recognition of the importance of the physical sciences, particularly chemistry, and in more recent times of biology, as represented in biochemistry, molecular biology and related fields, in medicine. They now saw a need to recognize the present and growing potential contribution of the behavioral sciences to medicine. This includes not only the biotropic aspects such as physiological psychology and individual psychology generally, but also the sociotropic aspects including social psychology, sociology and anthropology. For some, the medical curriculum should also include certain aspects of political science, economics and history.

The third group largely emphasized an approach. They argued that before discussing either one of the two topics just mentioned, it was important to redefine the position of the medical school in the total university setting. They maintained that the medical school had tended to become a quite independent and separate, as well as isolated, institution, and that it is important for medicine to return to the university of which it is a part. Their belief was that only from such a broadened setting could the behavioral sciences adequately be integrated into the medical program.

It is also in this same general context that Judge Bazelon's concern was presented. He indicated that he had been much disturbed by repeated experiences in calling upon psychiatrists for help to deal with the problems that came before him. He said he found psychiatrists inadequately prepared to deal with the social issues involved in the cases presented for his consideration. Not only were they limited in knowledge in this respect, but he felt also that they tended to report their findings in a jargonist fashion and were defensive about making available the information they had about patients in a clear and forthright manner. Although it is possible that the point was never explicitly made, I believe that implicit in what he was saying was the need for medicine to have a much greater social orientation, with the further implication that psychiatry particularly would inevitably benefit from this.

In the course of the meeting, two additional notions seemed to develop about what people expected to get from the Conference. At first the discussion seemed to be centered largely on determining what actually was to be the specific topic of the Conference. Although this was not decided, I believe that I am accurately reflecting the state of opinion at the time I left.

It may have been the difficulties in reaching some consensus on this topic that led to the development of an attitude that accepted a much less ambitious goal. This goal was that at the least the members of the Conference could mutually educate each other and go away with considerable gain for having attended. This mutual education could be of two major kinds. *1.* Being thrown together, antipsychiatrist and psychiatrist would be afforded opportunities to discuss frankly their attitudes toward each other and the failings they saw in each other. *2.* Another major group of contenders, the psychoanalytically oriented among the psychiatrists and the nonpsychoanalytically oriented (these included both organic and socially oriented psychiatrists), could confront one another in a similar manner. Although these two controversies are somewhat intertwined, in general they can be separated as I have described them. In addition, there were a few less important issues.

Since I, myself, was not primarily interested in contributing to this mutual education—I had been through this too many times in the past—it seemed wiser for me to withdraw and send in a separate statement to the Conference.

Humanizing the Physician

My interpretation of the major goal of the Conference was to contribute to the consideration of ways of achieving a greater humanization of the physician in the process of his medical education. I therefore limit my discussion to some aspects of this problem to which I feel my own background can contribute.

In addition to his substantive knowledge of basic medicine, certain characteristics describe the psychosocially oriented physician. Foremost among these is the recognition of the importance of *attitudes* in interpersonal relationships. Without the central acceptance of the all-importance of the patient and *his* attitudes, integral to which is the possession by the physician himself of a warm but objective approach toward patients, a physician would find it difficult to function optimally.

Besides this characteristic, the physician should have integrated into his approach to professional problems some degree of acceptance of a combination of the following five principles that underlie the understanding of personality: *1.* the *genetic* principle, which acknowledges the importance of antecedents in the genetic development to account for present manifestations of personality; *2.* the recognition of the *cryptic*, of unconscious and preconscious factors, as crucial determiners of behavior, the recognition that behavior has underlying motivations rarely perceptible to the actor, and frequently not even to the trained observer except with the use of special techniques; *3.* the *dynamic* notion that behavior is drive-determined, that beneath behavior ultimately lie certain innate or acquired drives; *4.* the general *psychobiological* assumption that the personality is integral and indivisible, that there is a pervasive interrelationship between psyche and soma—this involves the acceptance of an organismic principle of total rather than segmental personality; *5.* the *psychosocial* principle, which recognizes the integration of the individual and his environment as a unit, which recognizes that drives and their derivatives are expressed in individual response within a social context, and that the social is of equal importance with the individual in the determination of behavior.

Principles of Teaching

With these general principles as the broad goals of the teaching program, I shall consider briefly some specific aspects of this program, which fall more into my own area of competence, under four simple headings: to teach *what, how, when,* and *whom.*

We can consider the topic of *what* under two headings: what kind of material and what kinds of techniques to use. We are agreed that as much of the teaching as possible should use case material and come from *direct* contact with patients. It is necessary to present this material at the appropriate level of simplicity for the student's current state of knowledge. This calls for a proper combination of simplicity and complexity. Thus when cases are presented, there ought to be a special effort made to keep the material relatively simple and, especially in the earlier period, to emphasize the *therapeutic* aspects of a problem, not merely the presentation of the data. (Too often in psychiatry, for instance, the case is presented as too difficult to deal with therapeutically, and the student is left with a feeling of therapeutic nihilism.) In addition, the material should be real, not fabricated for the occasion. Students are quite sensitive to the presentation of what they consider as sham material. As far as possible, too, the material should occur in a service setting where something useful is being done for the patient. This, of course, is related to the previous point. Moreover, in the earlier years of medical training there should be a serious effort to select problems relevant to the medical field. The new medical student has waited a long time to come face-to-face with medical problems and is highly oriented in this direction. It is therefore wise to take advantage of his interest.

As for the kinds of techniques to be taught, I will mention elsewhere in this presentation the need for training the subjects in four kinds of observation technique. Three of these have to do with patients and one revolves around the observer himself.

It is important to emphasize that as much of the teaching as possible should take place in a setting of responsibility and involvement with the patient, where the student does as much of the actual work himself as is feasible at his stage of development. It should be carried out in an atmosphere of warm concern for the patient. Yet a student must have an opportunity to make errors and correct them. Therefore, at least in part, he should have the possibility of working with situations that at first do not carry with them danger for the patient. He should also have opportunities to learn as much as possible through teaching, which is a most effective method of learning. This would presumably mean in the earlier years of the medical program the teaching of persons like nurses and technicians, and in the later years perhaps teaching medical students of less advanced status.

One general principle can be laid down: the teaching relating to cases should come as early as possible in his program, and during the program the emphasis should be on graduating the difficulty of the material which the student comes in contact with.

Although there may be occasions when the student should be placed entirely on his own, ordinarily he should work independently under preceptorial guidance appropriate to the stage of his development. In addition, it is important of course that he have the opportunity to observe models among his professors who *do* rather than merely *say*.

Humanizing the Physician's Training

The behavioral sciences, insofar as they are concerned with the observation of human beings, face some very special problems. Since they involve the observer as instrument—the observation of human beings by other human beings—the importance of *variability* must be recognized. There is marked inter- and intravariability in the observed, and there is an equally great variability of both kinds in observers. We shall come to a consideration of the different kinds of observation and the ways in which we can help to reduce, or at least understand, the variability. However, we should first take up a problem, which has arisen during the course of the meetings, that points up the difficulties we face.

I refer to a question put by Jerrold Zacharias to Sally Provence. He asked her whether there were studies on what happened when a child was approached by a physician with a needle in order to take some blood. The implicit assumption, which I read into the question, was that if there were studies of that kind then presumably one could partial out what the effect was of the procedure itself. The difficulty as I see it, however, is that there is really no *one* answer to the problem put by Zacharias. There are several different answers, depending on the kinds of persons involved, and even different answers for different times in the same person.

In passing, I might indicate that I have been particularly impressed with this problem of variability of response because of my long-time concern with schizophrenics, in whom variability is so pronounced. This is another area where we can learn from the pathological to which Douglas Bond has referred. I would go along with him particularly in the point he made about working with the pathological but always with a window onto the normal. To rephrase Bond in literary terms, what we want is "A Room with a View."

FOUR KINDS OF OBSERVATION—DESCRIPTION

Let us now consider the several kinds of observations for which the human being as observer has to be the instrument. After having discussed these different kinds of observation I shall continue with the consideration of how one trains and improves the observer as instrument. Four major types of observation are involved: objective observation, participant observation, subjective observation, and self-observation.

In *objective observation*, we refer to the observations made from the outside directed towards the careful description of the impact on the individual of internal and external forces—physical, psychological and social—that are making him behave in the way in which he does. These observations are "naturalistic," they are made from outside the situation which the patient is in. The observer here is not directly involved with the patient.

The second kind of observation, *participant observation*, implies a much more intimate relationship between the observer and the observed. They are both part of a group. The observer has both to evaluate himself as a participant in the group, be able to make evaluations that are separated from those connected with his participation in the group, and evaluate what the effect of the act of observing has on the observed and the observation. The group may be just two people—the patient and himself—as in the simplest form of this interaction, history-taking. Except for history-taking, it may be that situations of the participant observer are relatively infrequent in ordinary medical relationships. In the psychiatric setting it is most strikingly found in psychotherapy, where the psychotherapist is both observer and therapist. It is possible that some thera-peutic situations in medicine are of this kind.

The third kind of observation is an especially important one for medicine. It involves *subjective observation,* the attempt to empathize with the patient, to try to understand how the pa-tient feels both about himself and his illness.

The fourth kind is *self-observation,* the understanding by the observer of his own feelings and attitudes, sort of asking oneself what makes one tick. This would seem to be vital in medicine, if one is to be sensitive to the psychological and social aspects of the illness of others.

It is clear that what we are emphasizing throughout is tech-niques for learning by experiencing rather than learning from hearsay. Because of this real-life learning, dangers are inherent in these techniques of, on the one hand, disturbing the validity of the observation and, on the other, of developing self-con-sciousness and exaggerated introspectiveness. Such dangers de-serve careful and deliberate consideration.

FOUR KINDS OF OBSERVATION—IMPLEMENTATION

Before actually beginning to work in the diagnostic area, stu-dents should have a preliminary and fairly extensive period of training devoted to *naturalistic observation* and description, procedures on which diagnosis is fundamentally based. Because so much of medicine depends on the description of the com-plexities of behavior, feelings and symptoms, a portion of the time of the first year should be spent in training students in careful observation and report. For this purpose one-way screens, paired observers, and recording devices of both sound and visual types should be used in settings where individuals and groups are under observation in free and controlled situa-tions. Constant checking of observer's reports against each other, against supervisor's observations, and against the mechanical devices should be standard practice. It is important that a healthy respect for careful observation and report be developed in students who are going to work in a discipline where a good share of the time the major instrument, in both respects, is the observer himself. With regard to reporting, both in this con-nection and with diagnostic study, strictness and insistence on high standards of succinctness and accurate terminology are essential. A further argument for early training in observation is suggested by Wenkebach's statement, *"Das Wissen verdrängt das Sehen,"* which points up the dangers that inhere in the early acquisition of technical terms and how frequently such knowledge serves as a barrier to accurate observation of the conditions with which the student is concerned.

In *participant-observation* the inadequacies of naturalistic observation are multiplied, and reveal themselves in two particular ways: one in relation to the data, and the other with regard to the effect on what is observed itself.

Like any reported observations, the data are bound by the capacity of the human observer as a reporting instrument. No matter how good human beings may be as conceptualizers, they are markedly handicapped sensorially, mnemonically, and expressively as observers and reporters. Put simply, they are limited in how much they can grasp, in how much they can remember of what they do grasp, and in how much and how well they can report even the slight amount they have grasped and remembered. The situation of participant-observation places an even greater stricture on the data, because we are dependent on a participant-observer whose participation is special and likely to be extensive. Distortions, both of omission and commission, arising from this situation and the personality of the observer undoubtedly enter. It is for these reasons that techniques for training of the kind mentioned earlier need to be given special attention.

With regard to *subjective observation,* we are concerned with the empathic insight into the nature of another person's difficulties and characteristics. It goes without saying that such insight is an important part of the physician's armamentarium. How to achieve the skill of "emphatic understanding," in which the student can learn to alternate between the identification and the objectivity that is called for, is the goal of training in this area. For such purposes exercises in role-playing and psychodrama under expert guidance can be most productive.

An important aspect of the problem of the observer as instrument, which arises particularly in dealing with motivational questions, is the degree to which one's own biases, affects, and problems, frequently only different from the patient's in intensity, color the material provided by the patient. It has become obvious to those working in the clinical field that some kind of control of this source of error is necessary. Many in the behavioral sciences, from their more extended experience with this type of material, have accepted the principle of the need for *self-evaluation* as a prerequisite for their work.

Physicians in general would also be helped by some kind of self-evaluation. For most, short methods of self-evaluation are preferable. Whatever the form, training should include self-examination under the competent guidance of experienced persons.

Physicians can perhaps adopt from social work practice a procedure that has been found effective in achieving at least partial self-knowledge. We refer to their use of detailed case supervision of students. From a parallel contact with preceptors, similar gains may possibly be achieved.

More General Questions

Two questions of a more general nature are also relevant in this discussion of the humanizing of the physician. Although significantly related to the whole field of medical education, a discussion of the questions of models and of ethics seems peculiarly appropriate in the context of a discussion of the behavioral sciences.

The aspect of "models" with which I am here concerned is not that of theoretical models, but rather that of teachers who might serve as models. Because of the considerable emphasis placed on courses in our universities and professional schools, one tends to pay less attention to the vehicles through which these courses are taught. In the end, it is amazing how much more permanent an impact teachers have on students by what they *do* in the context of what they say, rather than by what they just have to say. The proper selection of professors who *do* can go a great way to achieving the aims with which this Conference is concerned.

In relation to the teaching of medical ethics, the same general principles hold. It is hard not to sympathize with Felix Frankfurter ("Felix Frankfurter Reminisces," page 19) when he says in his discussion of his training at the Harvard Law School:

There weren't any courses on ethics, but the place was permeated by ethical presuppositions and assumptions and standards. On the whole, to this day I am rather leery of explicit ethical instruction. It is something that you ought to breathe in. It was the quality of the feeling that dominated the place largely because of the dean, James Barr Ames. We had no course in ethics, but his course on the law of trusts and fiduciary relations was so much more compelling as a course in ethics than any formal course in ethics that I think ill of most courses in ethics.

Unfinished Business

I shall assume that this Swampscott Conference has selected the "Humanizing of the Physician's Training" as its major topic and can come to some reasonable closure on it. One other important and broader problem relating to the behavioral sciences (raised by various conferees) is still left for consideration. It can perhaps be dealt with by a Conference that considers the medical school as part of the total university (the problem placed before us so cogently by Ralph Wedgwood). Behavioral science could in this context be considered in both its aspects as a basic science for medicine, as well as in its applied aspects.

Many of us felt that although this wider topic was of paramount importance, the group of conferees assembled at Swampscott was not necessarily the one to consider it. Such a Conference, we felt, would have to have a different membership—not only the particular persons and the fields represented at Swampscott, but others connected with university education generally and from other areas of the behavioral sciences as well.

Such a Conference, dealing with the medical school in the university and society, and with the behavioral sciences in both, could, I believe, make a substantial contribution to the understanding of the broader problem of which the one to which our particular Conference was devoted was only a part.

Critical Appraisal and Exhortation— from Two Laymen

MESSRS. WHITTEMORE AND KATAN

I

W E HAVE HAD a great many big questions on our hands, as well as a number of proposals of ways to go about answering them. First, the questions.

What are the limits or boundaries of medical practice?
How do these boundaries get established?
What is a patient?
Relationship of Doctor to the Healthy and Sick Patient
Is it impersonal, as in
   a. person to questionnaire file?
   b. investigator to investigated?
   c. personal confidential dialogue between human beings?
How can medical practice be made more humane? and what can be done to ameliorate the effects of institutionalism and a consequently dehumanized routine on the humanity of medical practice?

How do we go about deciding what behavioral sciences are relevant to medical practice?
Assuming that we can agree, in a general way, on answers to the questions above (a *large* assumption), what can we do with medical education to make medical practice more effective? Specifically, where and how do the behavioral sciences impinge upon medical education?
What are the contents of a behavioral science discipline, and *How* do we integrate it into the actual medical curriculum?

II

In trying to answer such questions, we have been conditioned, inevitably, by our respective medical and educational roles. That is, each of us has begun with our own assumptions, which have tended to be wildly divergent from those of our neighbors. Here are some:

If medical practice is to be effective, it must not be a catchall. It must strive to preserve its disciplinary integrity. Guilds have faults, but they have virtues too.

The behavioral sciences are not innately more humane than any other intellectual discipline; hence to incorporate them into medical education and practice is a categorical, administrative procedure that has no immediate bearing on the need for more humanity, etc.

Education must not be confused with learning. Constructing new curricula is largely a game with courses and hours. To do so is to miss the point: that most education does not occur in school, even good school, and to add to our besetting vice: we overteach.

The educational system is wrong. Start over.

There are vacuums out there that the doctor must fill, since nobody else is doing so. Columbia Point.

Medicine has entirely too much social and psychological power already. It is digging its own Napoleonic or papist grave.

Most of the behavioral sciences are not respectable. Or are not sciences.

Most of the behavioral sciences are not medical business. To introduce them is to confuse the doctor's role as well as to distort our culture's image of a patient.

We have to roll with the punches. The role of medicine is determined by changing cultural needs and changing scientific knowledge, not by medical prescriptions about what medical education and practice ought to be. The behavioral sciences are here. What are we arguing about?

To let them in intelligently, we need to reorganize all of medical education and practice.

To let them in without fuss, we need simply to add a Department of Behavioral Science.

Adding is precisely what we must avoid. We've had too much adding already. The specialization or departmentalization of education and practice is at the heart of the difficulty in making medicine humane.

III

Of all these conflicting assumptions, the best that can be said is that they are difficult to dislodge even by the best arguments, and large meetings do not produce good argument. The worst that can be said is that our various contestants are permanently unshakable; no argument will do. It would seem, therefore, that we must think of ways to reduce the domain of argument, and to figure out some way of operating beyond argument.

The general contention of our Swampscott group, we feel, is already that behavioral sciences are a necessity to the development of medical students. The alternatives that remain to be settled are:

1. Shall we first delineate the contents of the new discipline, and decide on its departmental role in the actual medical structure? *or*

2. Shall we operate on the assumption that this new addition in the curriculum is *not* and *should not* be just any new technical subject related with or added to the future medical practice, but a fundamental science encompassing all professions concerned with the alarming dehumanization of our exploded society? Would this not impregnate and change the whole curriculum?

We favor the second alternative, and believe that it is the role of this conference to rise above the daily contingency of personnel problems, and to transcend the many and enriching personal experiences, so as to draw general guidelines of a much needed blueprint. This is what we mean by getting beyond argument.

It is in the nature of the blueprint itself (and the subsequent change of attitude of the professional towards his society) that complete overhaul of the much too institutionalized education has to take place. The overhaul is not likely to take place in a complete manner within the going institutions, because they are where the old arguments and old perspectives are. Hence we think it is desirable to think of any overhaul as experimental. The point would be to find persons who would address themselves, inside or outside institutional situations, to a variety of medical problems by first throwing away their disciplinary tags. This is hard, but it is the challenge of this meeting. The fundamental nature of behavioral science is hopefully going to create an intimate as well as simultaneous interaction between itself and medical education. Behavioral science has direct bearing on the new perspectives we are looking for, in that it may well determine the character of the new professional.

References

1. Cope, Oliver, and Zacharias, Jerrold: Medical Education Reconsidered: Report of the Endicott House Summer Study on Medical Education, July, 1965, Philadelphia, Lippincott, 1966.

2. Coggeshall, Lowell T.: Planning for Medical Progress through Education, Evanston, Assn Amer Colleges, 1965.

3. Report on an Exploratory Conference: The Crisis in Medical Services and Medical Education, Fort Lauderdale, Florida, Feb. 20-25, 1966, sponsored by Commonwealth Fund and Carnegie Corporation, New York.

4. Report of the Citizens Commission: The Graduate Education of Physicians, Millis, John S., Chairman, 1966.

5. Aring, Charles: Intimations of Mortality: An Appreciation of Death and Dying, Lecture, Western Reserve, September, 1966.

6. Gross, Martin L.: The Doctors, New York, Random House, 1966.

7. Trendelenburg, Paul: Die Hormone ihre Physiologie und Pharmakologie, Berlin, Springer, 1934.

8. Fisher, C., Ingram, W. R., and Ransom, S. W.: The relation of the hypothalamico-hypophyseal system to diabetes insipidus, Arch Neurol Psychiat (Chic) *34*:124, 1935.

9. Hill, M., and Parkes, A. S.: Studies on the hypophysectomised ferret. III. Effect of post-coitus hypophysectomy on ovulation and the development of the corpus luteum, Proc Roy Soc *112*:153, 1932.

10. Sturgis, Somers H.: The Gynecological Patient, New York, Grune, 1962.

11. Harris, G. W.: The function of the pituitary stalk, Bull Hopkins Hosp *97*:358, 1955.

12. Bajusz, E., and Jasmin, G., eds.: Major Problems in Neuroendocrinology, Baltimore, Williams & Wilkins, 1964.

13. Gorbman, Aubrey, ed.: Comparative Endocrinology, New York, Wiley, 1958.

14. Wislocki, George B., and King, Lester S.: The permeability of the hypophysis and hypothalamus to vital dyes, with a study of the hypophyseal vascular supply, Amer J Anat *58*:421, 1936.

15. Hume, David M., and Egdahl, Richard H.: The importance of the brain in the endocrine response to injury, Ann Surg *150*:697, 1959.

16. Gloor, P.: Amygdala, *in* Field, John, ed.: Handbook of Physiology, Section I, Neurophysiology, vol. 2, chap. 58, Washington (DC), Amer Physiol Soc, 1960, p. 1395.

17. Brady, Joseph V.: Ulcers in "executive" monkeys: An account of experiments in which psychological stress causes physiological ills, Sci Amer *199*:95, 1958.

137

18. Harrison, Timothy S., Silver, Daniel M., and Zuidema, George D.: Thyroid and adrenal medullary function in chronic "executive" monkeys, Endocrinology 78:685, 1966.

19. Lidz, T., and Whitehorn, J. C.: Psychiatric problems in thyroid clinic, JAMA 139:698, 1949.

20. Cope, Oliver, Harrison, Timothy S., Wang, Chiu-an, Maloof, Farahe, and Sifneos, Peter E.: Graves' disease a psychosomatic disorder of multiple factor origin: Recent experiences with psychiatric treatment, to be published.

21. Jouvet, M.: Neurophysiology of the states of sleep, Physiol Rev 47: 117, 1967.

22. Aserinsky, E., and Kleitman, N.: Two types of ocular motility occurring in sleep, J Appl Physiol 8:1, 1955.

23. Dement, W. C., and Kleitman, N.: The relation of eye movements during sleep to dream activity: An objective method for the study of dreaming, J Exp Psychol 53:339, 1957.

24. Mandell, Arnold J., and Mandell, Mary P.: Biochemical aspects of rapid eye movement sleep, Amer J Psychiat 122:391, 1965.

25. Shapiro, A., Goodenough, D. R., Biederman, I., and Stesler, I.: Dream recall and the physiology of sleep, J Appl Physiol 19:778, 1964.

26. Clemens, Samuel L.: The awful German language, in A Tramp Abroad, Appendix D, Hartford, Amer Pub, 1891, p. 610.

27. Tuchman, Barbara, W.: The historian's opportunity, Saturday Review, Feb. 25, 1967, p. 29.

28. Cousins, Norman: The environment of language, Saturday Review, April 8, 1967, p. 36.

29. Harris, G. W., and Donovan, B. T., eds.: The Pituitary Gland, Berkeley, Univ Calif Press, 1966.

Index of Personal Names

139

Index of Subjects

Adrenal cortical hyperplasia, 45
Ambulatory care, 116-117
Animal(s), care, experience from, 71; stress in, 43
Anthropology, 16
Anxiety, defenses against, 32
Attitude(s), 120, 126

Behavior, *see* Personality; 31, 49, 51, 71; study of, 110-119
Behavior examination, in patient record, 75
Behavioral science, *see* specific science, e.g., Psychiatry; attitudes toward, 15, 79, 103, 104; body of knowledge, 89, 99-101; definition, 6; departments of, 82-84, 88, 102-104; importance to medicine, 25-36, 48-50, 98-104, 123-124; in premedical curriculum, 81, 105, 108; teaching in medical school, 84-85, 99, 100, 102-103, 121, 135
Brain, control of all body functions by, 40-42

Case study method, 120, 121
Child(ren), delayed speech in, 118; dying, 27, 28
Child development, 116, 117
Coggeshall Report, 24
Communication, jargon in, 64; processes of, 99
Computer medicine, 78-79
Conditioning, autonomic, 49
Council on the Study of Human Behavior, 112, 113
Courses, interdisciplinary, 102; on ethics, 133; single-discipline, abolition of, 100
Crippling, behavior study on, 115
Crowding, influence of, 49
Cushing's disease, 45

Day-care center, for emotionally disturbed children, 115
Death, *see* Terminal illness; denial by patient, 29
Departments, in medical school, 82-84, 88
Deprivation phenomena, 49
Disease(s), emotional aspects of, 16, 38, 51, *see* Psychosomatic disease; prevention of, 99
Dream(s), analysis of, 57; attention to one's own, 73

Economics, medical, 109
Education, institutionalized, correction of, 136; learning versus, 134; medical, *see* Medical education; premedical, study of behavior in, 108, 112
Emotional factors, *see* Stress; in disease and patient care, 9, 11, 16, 26, 40, 44, 45
Emotional problems, of patients, understanding of, 72
Empathy, 77
Endicott House Summer Study, 17-18, 23, 81, 90
Endocrine system, control by brain, 41
Environment, integration of individual with, 126; physiological function and, 39; study of, 118-119
Ethics, course on, 133
Experience, development of, in patient care, 74-75; personal, in medicine, 70-79

Faculty(ies), advice to, 80-91; as models, 107, 132; awareness of student adjustments, 107; inadequacy of, 85; in department of

141